What Your Doctor May *Not* Tell You About®

CHILDREN'S VACCINATIONS

STEPHANIE CAVE, M.D., F.A.A.F.P.
WITH
DEBORAH MITCHELL

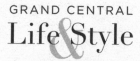

GRAND CENTRAL
Life & Style

NEW YORK · BOSTON

This book is not intended as a substitute for medical advice of physicians. The reader should regularly consult a physician in all matters relating to his or her health, and particularly in respect of any symptoms that may require diagnosis or medical attention.

Grand Central Life & Style
Hachette Book Group
1290 Avenue of the Americas
New York, NY 10104

www.GrandCentralLifeandStyle.com

Printed in the United States of America

RRD-IN

First revised edition: March 2010
10   9   8   7   6

Grand Central Life & Style is an imprint of Grand Central Publishing.
The Grand Central Life & Style name and logo are trademarks of Hachette Book Group, Inc.

The Hachette Speakers Bureau provides a wide range of authors for speaking events. To find out more, go to www.hachettespeakersbureau.com or call (866) 376-6591.

The publisher is not responsible for websites (or their content) that are not owned by the publisher.

Library of Congress Control Number: 2009927701

ISBN: 978-0-446-55571-5 (pbk.)

Author's Note

The information contained in this book is not intended to be a substitute for medical care and advice. You are advised to consult regularly with your physician about matters relating to your health (or with your pediatrician regarding matters relating to your child's health), including matters that may affect decisions as to whether, when, and in what form to administer vaccinations. In particular, if you are pregnant or have any other special condition requiring medical attention, you should consult with your physician.

This book is sold with the understanding that the author and publisher are not engaged in rendering legal or other professional advice. Laws and practices often vary from state to state and at the federal level; if legal assistance is required, the services of an attorney should be sought.

The identities of some of the patients referred to in this book, and certain details about them, have been modified.

The information provided in this book is based upon sources that the authors believe to be reliable. All such information is current as of this writing.

This book is dedicated to my husband, Donald; my sons and their wives, Chris and Shannon, Michael and Amy, Patrick and Annah; my grandchildren, Ramsey, Logan, Brennan Lee, Liam, Frances, Amelia, Ethan, Louisa, Walker, and Hudson Rae; and to all the precious children in the autism spectrum and their families, who hold a special place in my heart.

Acknowledgments

I wish to express my gratitude to all of my staff who have worked endless hours in the care of the children in our practice. I also want to thank my family, colleagues, and friends who have encouraged me to complete this book, Deborah Mitchell for her determination and dedication in the process of preparing the text, and Father Mario Termini, now deceased, who sustained us with his prayers.

I also wish to express my sincere gratitude to Barbara Loe Fisher for her help in obtaining information vital to the manuscript; and to Dr. Bernard Rimland, now deceased, who started the quest for safer vaccines when he realized the possible connection for autistic children.

Finally, to Congressman Dan Burton, who has worked tirelessly to make vaccines safer for all children, I extend the gratitude of many parents and professionals.

Contents

Introduction

Back in the middle of the twentieth century, mass immunization sounded like a good idea: We had deadly childhood diseases, we were developing vaccines that could prevent them, therefore, let's immunize all children so they won't get those diseases. And to make sure all, or nearly all, children were immunized, we made the shots mandatory.

And as the number of polio cases declined dramatically until they were nearly nonexistent, and as the number of children with measles and mumps and diphtheria and whooping cough dropped lower and lower, doctors and parents and health officials nodded and said, *Job well done.*

But beginning in the early 1980s, some parents and medical experts in the United States and elsewhere around the world noticed what appeared to be a connection between serious adverse health effects, including death, and vaccines. As the years passed, more and more parents, doctors, and even government officials began to see an alarming increase in the number of children with autism, learning disabilities, attention deficit disorder, juvenile diabetes, rheumatoid arthritis, sudden infant death syndrome (SIDS), asthma, and other medical conditions.

Their suspicions grew, as did the number of vaccines given to children. Whether vaccines are completely or partially the cause of the health issues named, or whether they have no role at all, has not yet been determined scientifically, but one thing is definite:

Parents are concerned and confused about vaccines. That concern and confusion prompted many parents and dedicated medical professionals to raise their voices in protest against unsafe vaccines, and those voices have finally prodded health and government officials to take action. In 1986, Congress passed the National Childhood Vaccine Injury Compensation Act, which officially acknowledged that vaccine injuries and deaths are real.

As a family practice physician, I was prompted into action myself around 1997, as more and more autistic children showed up in my office. Although the children came from different social and family environments, their histories were the same in one frightening way: They had all been healthy and developing normally—physically, emotionally, and mentally—until age fifteen to eighteen months. Then, the parents reported, their once happy, friendly babies disappeared, as if their inner spark had gone out. Suddenly the children lost speech, would not maintain eye contact, were highly sensitive to touch and noise, and were intentionally injuring themselves. The parents were horrified and frightened. And I did not know what to tell them.

But then as I studied the medical charts, I realized that all the children had one thing in common: All of them had deteriorated within weeks of receiving several vaccines simultaneously. It was then that I began to document my cases and read about other similar instances reported by doctors around the world. I discovered that I was not witnessing an isolated pocket of cases where I practiced in Baton Rouge, Louisiana, but verifying a phenomenon that was happening around the globe.

When word got out that I was investigating the relationship between vaccinations and autism, I was inundated with phone calls, letters, and e-mails from the United States and overseas. Most of this correspondence was from parents—parents who were scared and wanted answers. I had none to give them . . . but I was determined to try.

Autism used to be a rare condition, affecting 1 out of 10,000 infants. Now in some states it is diagnosed in 1 out of every 150 children. Between 1992 and 1997, the incidence of autism increased more than 300 percent. Can these increases be blamed on better diagnostic testing or coincidence? I doubt it. But I needed to know the answer.

I've never considered myself to be a maverick or the type of person who goes looking for conspiracies. As a young girl in school, I loved science and medicine, and my fascination with these subjects carried over to Louisiana State University, where I majored in medical technology and then taught for eight years. Along the way I got married and had three sons . . . and also got a master's degree in clinical chemistry. Then at age thirty-six, I took the plunge: I enrolled in Louisiana State University Medical School and fulfilled my dream of being a doctor.

Now I find myself delving into the intriguing and disturbing world of vaccinations, and like the parents of autistic children who come to see me, I want answers, too. These parents did what they'd been told to do: They got their children vaccinated. If they'd had any concerns about vaccines, if they had heard or read about the reports of autism or other problems some children were experiencing, including seizures, muscle diseases, and brain inflammation (encephalitis), they were often told by their doctors that there was nothing to worry about, and that they should consider themselves lucky to be living in a time when vaccinations are available.

But a glaring bit of evidence indicating that that luck was going to run out came on October 23, 1999. A front-page story in the *New York Times* revealed that the rotavirus vaccine was being recalled because it had been linked to a painful and potentially deadly bowel obstruction. It was the first time a vaccine had been withdrawn from the market because of serious side effects. But will it be the last?

No one, myself included, is suggesting that we stop all vaccinations and return to the days when the United States was plagued with smallpox, polio, diphtheria, and whooping cough. However, I, along with a growing number of doctors, researchers, and medical professionals, believe we cannot turn a blind eye to the rise in chronic childhood medical conditions that parallels the increase in mandated vaccinations, which dramatically increased vaccination rates.

We also cannot ignore hospitalizations, injuries, deaths, and serious health problems following vaccinations that are reported to the federal Vaccine Adverse Events Reporting System (VAERS), an entity that records such adverse events. Unfortunately, it is common knowledge that less than 10 percent of all adverse events following vaccinations are reported to VAERS, which means that instead of the 12,000 to 14,000 reports of hospitalizations, injuries, and deaths made every year, there may be as many as 120,000 to 140,000.

Can such a huge number of serious health problems following vaccinations be ignored? Can they be dismissed with the standard answer parents get when they ask about vaccine safety: "Don't worry. Vaccines are safe"?

Parents do worry, and there are many indications that they have every reason to. So shouldn't parents be allowed to review the benefits and risks of a given vaccine and then decide whether the vaccine should be given to their child?

This question raises the issue of who has the right to decide what is an acceptable risk for a child—parents or the government and big business. Vaccine manufacturers, federal health officials, and doctors admit that all vaccines carry a risk of injury and death, but they also dismiss those concerns by saying that side effects are usually mild, that serious reactions are extremely rare, and that the risk of getting the disease is much greater than the chance of suffering a serious reaction.

Why are doctors and health officials afraid to let parents make decisions about their child's vaccinations? Some of them claim that many parents would then not vaccinate their children at all, which could lead to a reemergence of such deadly diseases as polio and whooping cough, perhaps resulting in epidemics that might kill tens of thousands of infants and children.

I think this reason is unrealistic. I believe that the vast majority of parents want safe, effective vaccines supported by reliable scientific research. They also want to know the truth about the vaccines they are considering, things like:

- Why newborns are given hepatitis B vaccine even though there is little risk of the disease for the child.
- Accurate incidences of side effects for all vaccines.
- Which vaccines can be delayed or eliminated.
- Whether combination vaccines such as MMR (measles, mumps, rubella) can be given individually.

Parents are usually told the benefits of vaccines, but what about the risks or other unpleasant facts? Here are a few things you may not know about vaccines:

- Some vaccines contain poisons such as mercury, aluminum, and formaldehyde.
- In 1998, the French government suspended school-based vaccination programs giving hepatitis B vaccine to school-aged children because a case of multiple sclerosis was linked to the vaccine and more than six hundred cases of immune and neurological conditions were also reported.
- Some vaccines are made using human tissue from aborted fetuses.

- Many states require that by the time a child is five years old, he or she must receive more than forty-five doses of fourteen vaccines.
- Doctors report less than 10 percent of the adverse events associated with vaccines and/or occurring following vaccinations to the Vaccine Adverse Events Reporting System, charged with accumulating and tabulating these vaccine adverse events.
- In all states, parents can seek a medical waiver to exempt their child from mandated school vaccinations, and in some states they can also file a philosophical or religious exemption.

I'm not saying that doctors and others involved in the vaccine industry withhold information about vaccines because they don't care about children. But I do believe that part of the reason these individuals are afraid to let parents decide about vaccinations is economics: Vaccines are big business. The global vaccine market generates billions of dollars yearly for manufacturers.

There's much we don't know, but this much I am certain of: Parents who blindly listen to their doctors can no longer afford to do so. It's time for parents to ask questions and learn all they can about vaccines before a shot is scheduled.

It amazes me that since 2001, when this book was first published, the medical establishment has done very little to increase the safety and effectiveness of vaccines and stands behind a schedule that could prove to be detrimental to the immune systems of children. Thimerosal has been decreased in most vaccines and eliminated in others, but as of 2009 it remains in the influenza vaccine, which is recommended for use in six-month-old children and pregnant women.

The thimerosal is not considered a safety threat by the CDC, the Academy of Pediatrics, and the World Health Organization. Yet Thomas Burbacher, PhD, associate professor of environmental and occupation health sciences and director of the Infant Primate Research Laboratory at the University of Washington in Seattle, published a study in 2005 showing that in primates, ethyl mercury travels to the brain and stores as inorganic mercury. This form of mercury stays in the brain for a long period of time. While autism is touted to be purely genetic by many in the upper echelons of medicine, studies have shown it to be related to brain inflammation.

So what is the driving force that keeps so many brilliant people totally out of touch with the truth? Is it financial gain? What will happen to the future generations of children if we progress along the same paths that we have previously traveled? Will we keep injecting them with aluminum, mercury, MSG, human diploid cells, formaldehyde, unidentified viruses, and a host of other toxic substances while denying that we are contributing to their neurological demise?

This book represents part of my quest to get answers for myself and for parents. It is divided into three parts to make the journey easy. Part I discusses background and basic information about vaccines in general and some of the medical conditions associated with them. Chapter 1 explains the history of vaccines, what they are, how they work, and possible side effects. Chapter 2 explores vaccine safety, including how vaccines are tested, types of side effects, and ingredients found in vaccines. In chapter 3, you will learn about the controversy surrounding the use of mercury (thimerosal) in vaccines and how concerned individuals are working to get it removed from all vaccines. Chapters 4 and 5 discuss the most common medical conditions associated with recommended vaccine use, including autism and other neurological disorders such as learning disabilities and attention deficit disorder; and autoimmune disorders, including diabetes, asthma, rheumatoid arthritis, and others.

Part II consists of fourteen chapters. Chapters 6 through 17 explore each of the recommended vaccines individually: hepatitis B, DTP/DTaP (diphtheria, tetanus, pertussis), Hib, polio, MMR (measles, mumps, rubella), varicella (chicken pox), hepatitis A, pneumococcal, meningitis, influenza, rotavirus, and HPV (human papilloma virus). Each chapter explains the benefits and risks of the vaccine, the disease(s) it is designed to prevent, the side effects, who should and should not get the vaccine, and unique features, risks, or other information about the vaccine.

Chapter 18 discusses vaccines required for world travel. Chapter 19 introduces you to the vaccines of the future—those currently under development, some of which are slated for children. These include vaccines for cancer, as well as edible vaccines.

Part III provides some tools for parents. Chapter 20 explains parents' rights, including information about a nationwide registry that tracks children's medical (and vaccine) history, and how parents can apply for medical, religious, and philosophical exemptions. Chapter 21 provides parents with checklists of questions to ask themselves before their child gets a vaccine, questions to ask the doctor before a vaccine is given, and steps parents can take to modify reactions to vaccines. The final chapter covers the Vaccine Adverse Events Reporting System, which provides information on how to report an adverse event and how to apply for compensation if a child is injured by a vaccine.

For ease of reference, some information is repeated throughout the book. Consult with your doctor, and don't skip chapter 21—specifically the precautions that can be taken when you vaccinate your child. There are things you can do the day before, the day of, and the day after your child's vaccination that may help to make the experience a safer one for the child.

Some vaccines have accomplished what they were designed to do. But we must acknowledge certain realities about those vaccines when it comes to safety and effectiveness. All children deserve a healthy, safe childhood, and parents should be allowed to make informed decisions about their children's vaccine needs. I pray that this book helps parents make those decisions and leads them to other reliable sources in their search for the truth about vaccines as more research and information become available.

Part I

❀

INTRODUCING VACCINES

Chapter 1

❁

The Story of Vaccines

PERHAPS YOU'VE SEEN THE BUMPER STICKERS THAT SAY QUESTION AUTHORITY. Well, that's what's happening today with the increasing number of parents who are questioning the safety, the effectiveness, and even the necessity of the vaccines being given to their children and required by state law. Parents—and perhaps you are one of them—are questioning health care providers, state health officials, and one another about vaccinations. They are forming and joining action groups so they can learn more, and do more, about vaccine policies in the United States.

Next to the QUESTION AUTHORITY sticker should be another one that says KNOWLEDGE IS POWER. It's not a good idea to question authority when you don't know what you're talking about, because it won't help you accomplish your goals. And when the goals are safe health care and a healthy life for your children, the stakes are too high for you to miss the mark.

This chapter introduces you to the information you'll need to help you understand the world of vaccines and how they can affect you and your children. It explains what vaccines are, types of vaccines, how they are developed, and how they affect the immune system. You will also learn the answer to the question *Do I have to vaccinate my child?* as well as how to use the rest of this book to answer this question for each of the vaccines required by law and for those that are not.

FIFTEEN VACCINES . . . AND COUNTING

Today's parents are primarily concerned about the fifteen vaccines now recommended by the federal government. And there are dozens of other vaccines on the horizon, a future you may need to consider if you are a parent or grandparent. These other vaccines are covered in subsequent chapters. For now, however, here are the ones that are recommended in most states and mandated in some states:

Hepatitis B—the first vaccine children are typically given
DTaP—diphtheria, tetanus, pertussis (whooping cough), which is the newer form of the DPT (DTP) vaccine (see chapter 7 for details)
Hib—*Haemophilus influenzae* type B
Polio—the inactivated polio vaccine, or IPV, is the injected form of the polio vaccine, which as of January 1, 2000, was recommended over the oral polio vaccine (OPV) (see following and chapter 9 for more details)
MMR—measles, mumps, and rubella combination vaccine
Varicella—chicken pox
Hepatitis A
Pneumococcus
Rotavirus
Meningitis
HPV (human papilloma virus)

WHAT IS A VACCINE?

A vaccine is a substance that attempts to protect people against disease. To do that, vaccines are made from the virus or other pathogen (germ) that causes the disease the vaccine is designed to fight. You might say a vaccine uses fire to fight fire: A little bit of the pathogen is specially prepared and usually injected into the body so it can help fight off any "wild," or naturally acquired, versions of the disease. The purpose of that fight is to develop immunity.

The body has a complex system, called the immune system, that has procedures for producing and maintaining immunity. In short, when you get, say, a cold or flu virus or a bacterial infection, your body responds by producing substances called antibodies, minute protein molecules that fight against (anti) the foreign bodies (the viruses or bacteria). When you recover from the illness, your body retains some of those antibodies so it is ready to fight off the infection should it appear again. This is called immunity.

TWO TYPES OF IMMUNITY

Natural

Natural immunity is gained when viruses or bacteria enter the body, cause a disease, and the disease progresses normally. During the disease process, the body produces antibodies and disease-fighting cells, resulting in a natural immunity that is usually permanent.

When a child is naturally exposed to, say, the measles, the immune system responds immediately. Various immune cells begin to attack and eliminate the invading pathogens and send signals to other cells in the system, triggering them into action. Depending on the strength of the immune system, the body will reduce or even eliminate the disease before the symptoms show. In fact, experts have shown that the frequency of asymptomatic (having no symptoms of disease) infections outnumber clinical illnesses by at least a hundredfold, simply because the immune system has tremendous natural abilities to fight disease.

Vaccinated

Vaccinated immunity is artificial and often temporary. When the vaccines are injected into the body, they bypass many of the body's natural defenses. In a sense, the vaccine, along with the toxic additives in the solution, is thrust into the body unannounced. This "surprise" forces the body to overcompensate by producing more disease-fighting cells than it would if the infection were natural. This overstresses the body in two ways—it not only overproduces immune system cells but must also fight the infection (introduced by the vaccine), along with the chemicals and other additives in the vaccine. (These additives are discussed in chapter 2.)

Which is better, natural or vaccinated immunity? The answer may be a little of both. In any case, in order to find out, the least we (parents, researchers, medical professionals, lawmakers) should do is take a close look at the current vaccination schedule, each of the vaccines, and the research on the pros and cons of arbitrarily vaccinating all children. Currently most children are subjected to vaccinations beginning at birth or at two months of age, long before the immune system is ready to even begin to respond. Is this practice safe or wise? Are there alternatives? I believe there are, and it is my hope that you will find some alternatives for yourself in this book.

The main purpose of a vaccine is to stimulate the formation of antibodies at a concentration high enough to stop the pathogen in its tracks, and thus prevent those who get the vaccine from getting the disease. As long as you maintain a certain concentration for a specific disease, you have immunity.

Vaccination is no guarantee that your child or you will not get the disease. A small amount of the infectious agent can get past the antibodies and cause individuals to experience some mild symptoms, or occasionally even worse effects of the disease. (More on this topic in subsequent chapters.) However, in most cases, the vaccine prevents more serious symptoms from occurring. An up-to-date list of the vaccines recommended by the US government can be seen at or downloaded from www.aap.org/family/parents/immunize.htm. An in-depth explanation of each of these vaccines can be found in chapters 6 through 17. Included in these explanations is the Vaccine Information Statement (VIS). A VIS is an information sheet, produced by the Centers for Disease Control and Prevention, which informs vaccine recipients or their parents or legal guardians about the benefits and risks of the vaccine. Doctors are required by law to distribute a VIS for all mandated childhood vaccines.

AN INFANT'S IMMUNE SYSTEM

Infants come into the world with antibodies they have gotten from their mother through the placenta. Infants who are breast-fed continue to receive many important antibodies in the colostrum (the thick, yellowish pre-milk that is secreted during the first few days after a woman gives birth) and breast milk. Commercial infant formulas, although inferior to mother's milk, also provide essential nutrients for infants' health.

During the first year of life, the immunity an infant gets from its mother at birth wears off. To help boost the fading ability to fight certain diseases, vaccines are given. The idea behind vaccines is to provide just enough of the disease-causing substance to trick the body into producing antibodies against it. Once the antibodies are produced, they stay around, protecting the child against the disease they were designed to fight. Some vaccines provide this protection for life after just one or two shots; others require additional boosts of immunity.

The problem many doctors and parents have with vaccines given during the first few months of life is that an infant's immune system cannot adequately respond to a vaccine until he or she is four to six months old. I believe we need to look not only at the timing of these vaccinations—when they are given and how many are given at one time—but also at the ingredients in them and the dangers they may pose.

WANTED: DEAD OR ALIVE?

Vaccines have traditionally come in two basic forms: dead (inactivated or killed) and live. The vast majority of both forms are delivered one of two ways: via injection under the skin (subcutaneous) or into the muscle (intramuscular). (Polio and typhoid vaccines are also available in oral form.) In some cases, both live and killed vaccines are available to treat the same disease.

A third type of vaccine, the recombinant DNA vaccine, is

the product of genetic engineering. It is the newest form, but there are questions about safety and efficacy.

Live Vaccines

Live vaccines are made in a laboratory from the living organism (usually a virus) that causes the disease. Live vaccines are attenuated, or weakened, so they will cause the body's immune system to generate an immune response without (hopefully) causing the disease. Some people, however, do respond to a vaccination by developing symptoms of the disease, although in most cases they are mild. Examples of live attenuated virus include polio (oral), measles, mumps, chicken pox, rubella, influenza, rotavirus, HPV, and yellow fever. Live bacterial vaccines include one for typhoid fever and Bacillus-Calmette-Guerin (BCG) vaccine, which is used for tuberculosis.

Some experts claim that the immune system responds to live, attenuated vaccines the same way it does to a natural infection; others disagree (see "Two Types of Immunity," above). In fact, even proponents of live vaccines agree that live vaccines can cause a mild version of the disease they are designed to prevent. People who question the wisdom of giving live vaccines, especially to infants and young children, say these vaccines may have much more serious consequences, pointing to the correlation with autism and autoimmune diseases (see chapters 4 and 5).

Killed Vaccines

A killed, or inactivated, vaccine consists of all or part of the disease-causing organism that has been killed or rendered inactive. Unlike live vaccines, killed vaccines cannot reproduce, so they are not able to cause the disease they are designed to prevent. They trigger a weaker response by the immune system than do live vaccines. They also tend to be safer than live vaccines for people who have a weakened immune system, for pregnant women, and for children younger than one year.

Most killed vaccines are protein-based, like the bacteria they mimic. Some of these bacteria are coated with sugars called polysaccharides. When scientists tried to develop vaccines for sugar-coated bacteria, they found that pure polysaccharide vaccines didn't work well in infants. But when they joined (conjugated) the polysaccharide to a protein, the vaccines were much more effective for infants and young children.

Inactivated vaccines are used for the following diseases: cholera, hepatitis A, hepatitis B, influenza, pertussis (whooping cough), polio (injected), rabies, and typhoid.

Another type of inactivated vaccine is the toxoid. These vaccines are made by inactivating the toxins (poisons) produced by bacteria and viruses. The vaccines against diphtheria and tetanus are toxoids.

Recombinant DNA Vaccines

Another type of vaccine is a recombinant DNA (genetically engineered) vaccine. The hepatitis B vaccine is one example. Rather than using the entire organism, recombinant DNA vaccines are made by taking specific genes from the infectious agent (viruses or bacteria) and adding them to the vaccine culture. For example, hepatitis B vaccine is made by inserting a portion of the hepatitis B virus gene into baker's yeast, the culture in which this vaccine is produced.

Experts say recombinant DNA vaccines are more effective and safer than other types of vaccines because they don't contain the entire infectious agent and thus cannot cause an actual infection. However, the greatest concern about recombinant DNA vaccines is that they may cause the immune system to produce antibodies, which in turn attack parts of the body and cause health problems. Much is still unknown about the effects of recombinant DNA vaccines.

ONE SHOT, TWO SHOTS, THREE SHOTS, FOUR?

It would be nice if we could protect children against all threats of childhood diseases, such as chicken pox, measles, diphtheria, whooping cough, and polio, in one strategically administered—and completely safe—shot or pill. Unfortunately, that is not the case. In fact, children receive more than forty-five doses of fourteen vaccinations by the age of five years. Not only do children need a separate vaccine for most diseases (hepatitis B, polio, Hib, and chicken pox are single vaccines; DTaP and MMR are multiple), they also need more than one dose of most vaccines. The one or more additional doses of a vaccine given to help ensure the protection provided by the original dose(s) are called boosters. Booster doses are given a few months or sometimes years after the original dose. For example, the first three DTaP shots are the original doses given to establish immunity. The next two shots at twelve to eighteen months and at four to six years are boosters, as is the recommended Tdap for adolescents.

Are Boosters Necessary?

To determine whether children need a booster, doctors can check their titers—the measurement of the amount or concentration of a substance in a solution. In the case of vaccines, it refers to the amount of antibodies present in patients' blood and serum. If the antibody titer is high enough to make them immune to specific diseases, they may not need a booster. Researchers are finding that some of the vaccines routinely given do actually confer immunity for longer periods of time than was originally thought. Unfortunately, doctors don't usually check a person's titers before giving a booster. If the practice of checking titers were put into place, we would probably be able to eliminate some of the boosters now being given to our children, and thus reduce the risk of adverse effects. Parents can consider asking that titers be checked before a booster is given. The titers for measles, mumps, and rubella seem to be more reliable than others.

WHERE IT BEGAN:
A BRIEF HISTORY OF VACCINES

Vaccines are not a new idea, although the early forms would not be popular in today's world. One of the first recorded attempts at vaccine-like treatments occurred sometime during the seventh century when a group of Buddhists decided they could become immune to the effects of snake venom by drinking the foul substance. In sixteenth-century China, writings describe how people were inoculated against smallpox by placing the powdered scabs from infected children into the noses of healthy children. These people had the right idea—they realized they could help prevent a disease or condition by exposing themselves to a form of the substance that caused it—but they didn't fully understand what they were doing at the time.

A more scientific approach was used in the late eighteenth century by Edward Jenner, who discovered that inoculating people with the animal disease cowpox made them immune to the deadly human disease smallpox. This was an interesting concept, and fortunately for Jenner it helped save lives, but the use of an animal disease to treat humans also presented the possibility that other diseases could be introduced along with the intended virus. Another approach was needed.

Between the time Jenner published his work in 1798 and Louis Pasteur developed the first rabies vaccine for humans in 1885, several scientists, including Pasteur, were investigating this problem. During that time, Pasteur enhanced the concept of attenuation, which is the use of a weakened form of a virus to provide immunity. Pasteur found that a weakened form of chicken cholera (an attenuated form) was highly effective in preventing the disease. Attenuated vaccines are widely used today.

Protests against the use of vaccines are nothing new. When Pasteur introduced his rabies vaccine for humans in 1885, both doctors and the public rallied against its use. At the turn of the century, British troops fighting in the Boer War in South Africa strongly protested being inoculated against the serious disease typhoid.

Many exciting events and discoveries occurred in the world of vaccines in the decades that followed (see "Milestones in Vaccine Development and Use," below). Perhaps the biggest boon to the immunization movement was the development of polio vaccines, one by Jonas Salk and the other by Albert Sabin. The fear of polio by the public was so great that mass immunization with Salk's injectable vaccine beginning in 1955 was welcomed with open arms. Salk's vaccine could not provide complete protection against all three polio viruses, so Sabin's live oral vaccine—introduced in 1961 and offering broader immunity—quickly became the more commonly used. The oral vaccine is no longer recommended because it's been proven to actually cause polio in some recipients and in the close contacts of those recently vaccinated.

History is still being made. New vaccines and new formulations of existing vaccines are being developed all the time. Chapter 19 looks at some of the vaccines on the horizon.

MILESTONES IN VACCINE DEVELOPMENT AND USE

1906: Vaccine against whooping cough (pertussis) developed.

1921–1928: Vaccine against diphtheria developed.

1933: Tetanus vaccine available.

1940s: Combination diphtheria, tetanus, and pertussis (DTP) vaccine developed.

1946: DTP vaccine available.

1954: Jonas Salk develops first polio vaccine (injectable) in the United States.

1955: Polio vaccine is licensed and distributed free through the Poliomyelitis Vaccination Assistance Act.

1963: Oral polio vaccine by Abert Sabin is licensed.

1963: Measles vaccine licensed.

1968: Mumps vaccine developed.

1969: Rubella vaccine licensed.

1978: Pneumococcal vaccine becomes available.

1979: MMR vaccine added to routine childhood vaccination schedule.

1981: Japan licenses DTaP vaccine, a safer version of the DTP vaccine.

1982: Hepatitis B vaccine becomes available. Parents of children who were injured by the DPT vaccine form Dissatisfied Parents Together (later to evolve into the National Vaccine Information Center) to lobby for safer pertussis vaccine in DPT shots.

1986: First recombinant hepatitis B vaccine licensed. Congress passes the National Childhood Vaccine Injury Act.

1987: Hemophilus influenza type B (Hib) vaccine licensed.

1991: The CDC recommends that all infants receive the

hepatitis B vaccine; the United States licenses DTaP vaccine for children eighteen months and older. The hepatitis B, Hib, and DTaP are given at the same visit for the first time.

1995: Varicella vaccine licensed.

1996: The FDA licenses safer DTaP vaccine for children under eighteen months old and the CDC's Advisory Committee on Immunization Policy (ACIP) recommends that the DTaP vaccine be used instead of the original DTP shot.

1998: The French government suspends hepatitis B vaccination programs in schools because of reports of multiple sclerosis and other immune and brain problems. Rotavirus vaccine approved for infants.

1999: The genetically engineered vaccine for rotavirus is removed from the market after many vaccinated infants become seriously ill with bowel blockage and at least one dies. Congressional hearings on vaccine safety begin. Manufacturers are asked to eliminate or significantly reduce the amount of mercury in vaccines.

2000: The CDC recommends using the injectable polio vaccine instead of the oral form because the latter caused up to ten cases of polio per year. A new pneumococcal vaccine—Prevnar—is recommended for infants.

2002: Lyme vaccine pulled off the market. Pentavalent (DTaP, hepatitis B, IPV) licensed. CDC recommends the influenza vaccine for children as young as six months of age.

2003: Smallpox vaccine recommended for first responders.

2005: Meningitis vaccine licensed.

2006: New rotavirus vaccine (RotaTeq) licensed.

2007: HPV (Gardasil) vaccine licensed.

DO I HAVE TO VACCINATE MY CHILD?

This question is being asked more and more often by parents as they hear and read about the association between vaccines and various serious health conditions. Although there are no federal mandates that force parents to have their children vaccinated, state laws essentially act as such. Many parents are unaware that they can get an exemption from vaccinating their child for medical, philosophical, or religious reasons, depending on the laws of their particular state. An explanation of state laws and exemptions and how to get them is found in chapter 20.

If a child does not meet state vaccination requirements, goes to school, and the truth is discovered, the school can have the child removed. There have also been instances in which state officials have charged parents with neglect for failing to vaccinate children with all mandated vaccines.

Before parents make decisions not to vaccinate a child and deal with the consequences, they need to have full access to information that allows them to weigh the risks and benefits of the growing number of recommended vaccines. Parents need to know that there are legal avenues they can take to exempt their children from receiving vaccinations.

PROGRAMS THAT PROTECT CHILDREN

As parents and physicians have seen an increasing number of injuries associated with vaccinations, government and private-sector organizations have formed to ensure that children harmed by vaccines will receive some compensation and that parents have access to all available information about the pros and cons of vaccination. There are dozens of such groups and programs, but some of the main ones designed to help protect our children include:

- National Vaccine Information Center (NVIC)
- National Childhood Vaccine Injury Compensation Program
- Vaccine Adverse Events Reporting System (VAERS)

Details about these organizations and others and the services they provide are discussed throughout this book, and there is a list in the appendix.

BOTTOM LINE

We are fortunate that we have stopped the epidemics of smallpox, polio, diphtheria, and measles. Vaccines have become a part of our world—for the current health of our children and for future generations. But because each act of administering small bits of disease and foreign substances to children opens the door to the possibility of debilitating consequences or even death, every possible attempt must be made to ensure that today's vaccines and those in the future are as safe as possible.

I am not suggesting that we return to the days without vaccines. But we must seriously address what appears to be an obvious link between the epidemic of developmental delays and autoimmune diseases, and the increasing number of mandatory vaccines. All parents should know the advantages as well as the dangers associated with every vaccine, every time it is given. They should know the positive and negative consequences of refusing to have their children vaccinated, and be made aware of how they can go about getting exemptions. And the government, industry, health care professionals, and parents must band together to get the research needed to determine the safety of these vaccines. The stakes are too high for us to do otherwise.

NOTES

Ad Hoc Group for the Study of Pertussis Vaccines. *Lancet* 1 (1988): 955–60.

Blennow, M., and M. Granstrom. "Adverse Reactions and Serologic Response to a Booster Dose of Acellular Pertussis Vaccine in Children Immunized with Acellular or Whole-Cell Vaccine as Infants." *Pediatrics* 84 (1989): 62–67.

Diodati, Catherine J. M. *Immunization: History, Ethics, Law and Health.* Ontario, Canada: Integral Aspects, 1999, 50 passim.

The Group on Immunization Education of the Society of Teachers of Family Medicine Web site: www.immunizationed.org.

The Journal of Family Practice Web site: www.jfponline.com.

National Institute of Molecular Biology and Biotechnology, at www .upd.edu.ph/~mbb/. Information on recombinant DNA vaccines.

Saroso, J. S., et al. "A Controlled Field Trial of Plain and Aluminum Hydroxide–Absorbed Cholera Vaccines in Surabaya, Indonesia, During 1973–75." *Bulletin of the World Health Organization* 56 (1978): 619.

"Vaccines Across the Life Span." *Journal of Family Practice,* February 2007.

World Health Organization Web site: www.who.int/vaccine-diseases/ safety/parents.

Chapter 2

❊

How Safe Are Vaccines?

Wヘン IT COMES TO VACCINES, THE BIG QUESTION IS: *How safe are they?* The answer is both simple and complex. While choosing to refuse all vaccinations for your children may expose them to serious health risks, blindly accepting all vaccines without question and according to the proposed schedule may also have grave consequences.

There are benefits and risks associated with every vaccine, and I believe it is your right to know both sides and the controversies that surround every vaccine. One goal of this book is to provide you with the most up-to-date information on each vaccine now mandated for children, as well as vaccines on the horizon, so you can decide for yourself what is best for your children.

There are many theories about how vaccines may cause harm. For more than two decades, there have been intense discussions at local, state, and federal levels regarding possible links between immunization and various physical and emotional/psychological problems, such as those discussed in chapters 4 and 5. The adverse effects of vaccines appear to be mild and temporary in many cases, but certainly not in all of them. Until we are able to assess what vaccines are doing to the human body at a cellular level, we will never know the full impact they have on the health of our children.

This chapter explores vaccine safety. It looks at the types of reactions people have to vaccines, how vaccines are tested, multiple dosing, how vaccines are made, ingredients in vaccines, and the story of a vaccine gone bad: the rotavirus vaccine.

MASS IMMUNIZATION AND HERD IMMUNITY

In many parts of the world, including the United States, there are programs for mass vaccination of different populations. In the US, the primary targets are infants and young children, whose parents are told they should receive multiple doses of fourteen different vaccines between birth and the age of five. The rationale behind mass vaccination was stated by the thirteenth World Health Assembly: "Vaccination is not simply a personal affair. Indeed, it is essentially a community matter, since the objective of most vaccination programmes is to produce a herd immunity."

Herd immunity is the level at which a certain population can resist disease. To achieve a high level of herd immunity, advocates of mass immunization strive for the highest vaccination rates possible with the hope that virtually everyone in the selected group will be protected from disease.

One of the main arguments of those who oppose mass vaccination of children is that government entities, vaccine manufacturers, and other players in the pro-mandatory-vaccine arena have a dangerous one-size-fits-all attitude. Yet every child is an individual, with a unique genetic makeup, social environment, and family and personal medical history that can have an effect on how he or she will react to a vaccine. Nor are all diseases and vaccines the same. Vaccines can save, and they can harm. The line between the two may be fine at times, but it is a line we must clearly define because lives are at stake.

TYPES OF ADVERSE REACTIONS

While an explanation of the dangers of each vaccine can be found in its respective chapter (chapters 6 through 17), there are some general types of adverse effects, injuries, and complications that are associated with vaccinations. Some occur almost immediately after a child receives the injection; others may take hours, days, or even months to appear.

Toxic

In vaccines that contain killed bacteria, the bacteria can release toxins into the bloodstream. If these toxins reach the brain, neurological problems, including autism, ADD, and behavioral problems can develop. Autism and related disorders are discussed in chapter 4.

Autoimmune

Vaccines are supposed to trigger the body's immune system to attack the vaccine's components. But what if the immune system attacks more than it is supposed to—say, a part of the body that is chemically similar to the vaccine? This type of reaction is called autoimmune, meaning that the body attacks itself (auto).

Such reactions have been reported for measles, tetanus, and flu vaccines, says Marcel Kinsbourne, M.D., a pediatric neurologist and research professor at the Center for Cognitive Studies at Tufts University. A review of the literature shows a possible link between type 1 diabetes and several vaccines. These include Hib, hepatitis B, rubella, and mumps. Dr. J. Barthelow Classen has analyzed vaccinations and disease incidence data from foreign countries and has conducted some research on mice and rats. He demonstrated that eight-week-old rats and mice injected with DPT vaccine had a higher incidence of diabetes than those that were not injected. This will be covered in detail in chapter 5.

Infectious

Vaccines that contain live viruses may cause the disease they are supposed to prevent. One example is the oral polio vaccine, which as of January 1, 2000, is no longer recommended for use because it was responsible for approximately ten reported cases of polio each year it was given. Also, measles, mumps, rubella, and chicken pox vaccines sometimes lead to symptoms of the diseases they were designed to prevent.

SAFE VACCINES: SCIENCE OR FICTION?

Doubting the safety and effectiveness of vaccines is not far-fetched. Not only are there tens of thousands of vaccine adverse events reported—but tens of thousands more go unreported. The pharmaceutical industry and medical field have a record of causing harm, as well as good, through the use of recommended, prescribed drugs, and vaccines.

This fact became glaringly apparent in April 1998, when an

article in the *Journal of the American Medical Association* reported that more than 2 million Americans become seriously ill and 106,000 die each year because of toxic reactions to drugs that were prescribed for them by health care professionals. Among children, vaccines and antibiotics are responsible for more negative reactions than any other prescribed drugs. I am not saying that drug companies and doctors intentionally harm people. But the reality is that no drug is safe for everyone, and some are much more dangerous than others.

In October 1999, Neal Halsey, M.D., director of the Institute for Vaccine Safety, Johns Hopkins University School of Public Health, testified before the US House of Representatives Committee on Government Reform. In his statement, he said: "Vaccine safety should be based on good science, not hypotheses, opinion, individual beliefs, or observations. Federal agencies responsible for vaccine safety and major universities have procedures to assure high-quality scientific research and reviews of vaccine safety issues." But many people question whether these procedures are being followed, especially given cases like the rotavirus vaccine, which was put on the market in 1998 and removed in 1999 after it caused nearly a hundred serious adverse reactions and at least one death. (See "Rotavirus Vaccine: An 'Experiment' Gone Bad" later in this chapter.)

Mass Immunization = More Illness

The truth is, there is much scientists don't know about how vaccines work in the body at a cellular and molecular level. Also lacking is an understanding of the long-term effects of continuing to mass-vaccinate our children. We do know that since the late 1950s, when mandatory mass vaccinations started in the United States, there has been an increase in the incidence of immune system and neurological disorders, including attention deficit disorder, asthma, autism, childhood diabetes, chronic fatigue syndrome, learning disabilities, rheumatoid arthritis, multiple sclerosis, and other chronic health problems.

"Rates of asthma and attention deficit disorder have doubled; diabetes and learning disability have tripled; and most states have experienced a 300 percent or more increase in autism," says Barbara Loe Fisher, cofounder and president of the National Vaccine Information Center, the largest and oldest national, nonprofit organization dedicated to the prevention of vaccine-related injuries and deaths. Are these increases just a coincidence or are they partly a result of better diagnostic testing? Or could it be, as many experts and parents believe, that these chronic health problems are the result, at least in part, of continued assaults on the immune systems of infants and young children with injections of viruses, bacteria, and various toxic substances?

"Best Available Science"

Officials with the Centers for Disease Control (CDC), the Food and Drug Administration (FDA), and the American Academy of Pediatrics (AAP)—three organizations involved in establishing vaccination policies—insist that vaccines are safe. In his testimony before the House Committee on Government Reform on August 3, 1999, Samuel L. Katz, M.D., of the AAP and the Infectious Diseases Society of America (IDSA), indicated that the appearance of these illnesses after vaccinations was a coincidence.

"We give vaccines in the first two years of life, when all of these disorders have their common onset, so that guilt by temporal association is very difficult to separate from guilt by causality," he said. He also assured his audience that there exists a "robust system of checks and balances" monitoring vaccine safety and that the procedures "reflect the best available science." These assurances, however, have not satisfied those who are concerned about vaccine safety, or those who must live with the consequences of vaccine-related disabilities.

Missing: Sufficient Testing of Vaccines

The tremendous increase in the number of reported and observed medical problems that are being associated with vaccinations by parents and medical professionals has sparked a movement in the United States and elsewhere in the world to demand more and better studies of the potential long-term or chronic adverse effects of vaccines. Ronald Kennedy, professor of microbiology and immunology at the University of Oklahoma, says, "The whole problem with vaccine adverse effects is that there are too many hypotheses without scientific support. We need to support careful scientific investigations in this area, but unfortunately the federal government and the pharmaceutical companies don't agree and don't support such efforts."

Howard Urnovitz, PhD, a microbiologist and founder of the Chronic Illness Research Foundation in Berkeley, California, argues that the federal government keeps insisting that "there's no scientific evidence to prove that vaccines cause chronic diseases, but they won't fund any research in that area either. If you don't look for something, you won't find it."

Genetic Predisposition

Ronald Kennedy believes that certain vaccines should not be given to people who have a family history of or predisposition for autoimmune disorders, such as rheumatoid arthritis and multiple sclerosis. Vaccine activists like Barbara Loe Fisher agree. She notes that there have been cases in which several children in the same family have been harmed by a specific vaccine, yet health officials still insist that the rest of the children be vaccinated and that the injured children get booster shots. Since 1982, Fisher has been urging the US government and vaccine manufacturers to investigate what these genetic predispositions may be and to urge those who administer vaccines to screen individuals for these tendencies. "The government has no business forcing vaccinations on these people . . . while refusing to do research to discover the genetic markers that would identify who is susceptible to adverse reactions," she says.

VACCINES:
RECIPES FOR SUCCESS OR DISASTER?

One safety issue that I believe is often overlooked when it comes to vaccines is the "recipe." All vaccines have three main types of ingredients: the "bug" material—killed or live viruses or bacteria, toxoids, or DNA; ingredients that are added to perform a variety of functions; and the culture in which the vaccines are prepared. The bug material is explained in chapter 1. Let's look at the other factors.

Added Ingredients

The recipe for the vaccines your child is taking may include the following ingredients:

- **Aluminum:** This metal is added to vaccines, in the form of gels or salts, to promote the production of antibodies. Aluminum has been named as a possible cause of seizures, Alzheimer's disease, brain damage, and dementia. A study published in *Pediatrics,* for example, found that children who received a pertussis vaccine containing aluminum experienced allergic responses while children who received a non-aluminum pertussis vaccine did not have such reactions. These results are supported by other studies published in *Lancet* and the *Bulletin of the World Health Organization.* Aluminum is used in the DTP, DTaP, and hepatitis B vaccines.

- **Benzethonium chloride:** The anthrax vaccine (given primarily to military personnel) contains this ingredient. It is a preservative and has not been evaluated for human consumption.

- **Ethylene glycol:** This is the main ingredient in antifreeze. It is used in some vaccines (for example, DTaP, polio, Hib, hepatitis B) as a preservative.

- **Formaldehyde:** This substance is of great concern because it is a known carcinogen (cancer-causing agent). Formaldehyde is perhaps best known for its use in the embalming process, but it is also used in fungicides, insecticides, and the manufacture of explosives and fabrics. It is considered to be incompatible with many other substances, including one that is also found in some vaccines—phenol. In vaccines, liquid formaldehyde, called formalin, is used to inactivate germs. Not only is formaldehyde toxic, but, according to Sir Graham S. Wilson, author of *The Hazards of Immunization,* it is also inadequate as a disinfectant. This fact has been known for decades, says Catherine J. M. Diodati, author of *Immunization: History, Ethics, Law and Health,* and the continued use of "this unreliable and hazardous substance clearly violates the principle of nonmaleficence [not doing harm]." Formaldehyde may be found in several vaccines. More recent research from scientists at Imperial College, London, shows that reactive groups called carbonyls are created after the formalin damages the proteins in the vaccines. This can trigger an autoimmune condition in which the body does not recognize itself. What results is damage to the body in many different systems. In the 1960s, carbonyls in the respiratory syncytial virus (RSV) vaccine "triggered a powerful immune response that caused severe side effects leading to hospitalization and several deaths."

- **Gelatin:** This known allergen is found in the varicella and MMR vaccines.
- **Glutamate:** Glutamate is used to stabilize some vaccines against heat, light, and other environmental conditions. It is known to cause adverse reactions and is found in the varicella vaccine.
- **Neomycin:** This antibiotic is used to prevent germs from growing in vaccine cultures. Neomycin causes allergic reactions in some people. It is found in the MMR and the polio (IPV) vaccines.
- **Phenol:** This coal-tar derivative is used in the production of dyes, disinfectants, plastics, preservatives, and germicides. It is highly poisonous in certain doses and actually harms rather than stimulates the immune system, which is the exact opposite of what vaccines are designed to do. Phenol is used in the preparation of some vaccines, including typhoid.
- **Streptomycin:** This antibiotic is known to cause allergic reactions in some people. It is found in both forms of the polio vaccine.
- **Thimerosal:** This substance is a preservative that contains nearly 50 percent ethyl mercury, which means it has many of the same properties mercury has—thus it is very toxic. For decades, it was used in many vaccines on the market. Most childhood vaccines now are offered in single doses, which are thimerosal-free. See chapter 3 for an in-depth look at this substance.

Although it is true that these ingredients are present in vaccines, they are, for the most part, poisons or known allergens. Once they are injected into your child's bloodstream and immature immune system, they are not adequately eliminated by the bile and the liver, because bile production has not yet matured. As one mother put it, "I wouldn't give my child food with MSG, and I certainly wouldn't feed him aluminum, mercury, or formaldehyde. So why would I knowingly have those things injected into his bloodstream?"

Vaccine Cultures: How Vaccines Are Made

What follows is a description of basic vaccine formulas. However, the recipes for vaccines are not all the same. Information on each individual vaccine is provided in the relevant chapters of part II.

For vaccines that are not genetically engineered (as are hepatitis B vaccine and many of the vaccines now under development), a toxic bacterium or a live virus is weakened (attenuated) by repeatedly passing it through a culture medium, such as human cells (aborted fetus tissue), monkey kidney tissue, chicken embryo, guinea pig embryo cells, or calf serum, to reduce the organism's potency.

Killed vaccines are inactivated using heat, radiation, or chemicals. The weakened virus or bacterium is then strengthened by adding stabilizers and adjuvants—substances that boost the antibody production in the vaccine such as those named under "Added Ingredients," above.

Dangers may be introduced during the making of vaccines. All viruses, dead and alive, contain DNA and RNA, the carriers of genetic material. When vaccines are made, these viruses are placed in a culture medium, which may include rabbit brain tissue, guinea pig tissue, dog kidney tissue, monkey kidney tissue, chicken embryo, or chicken or duck egg protein. The RNA and DNA from the viruses can be picked up by the animal cells in the culture. Cells in which the viral RNA integrates into the DNA of the animal cells are called pro-viruses.

Pro-viruses can stay dormant (inactive) in the body for many years. If they become active, many experts believe they are responsible for autoimmune disorders, in which the immune system cannot distinguish between its own tissues and foreign invaders, and so the body attacks itself. Examples of autoimmune diseases include diabetes, rheumatoid arthritis, and asthma, and are discussed in chapter 5. In addition, the animal proteins (tissue is composed of proteins) used in the cultures are not digested in the human body, and undigested proteins are a major cause of allergies. Undigested proteins can also attack the protective covering on the nerve cells and cause neurological problems.

The other kind of tissue in which some vaccines are grown is human fetal tissue. At least one of each of the available polio, MMR, rabies, chicken pox, and hepatitis A vaccines are made in this manner. The question about whether these vaccines can cause an autoimmune response once they are injected has not been definitively answered and deserves study. The use of human fetal tissue is also an ethical issue for some people, as the tissue has usually been obtained from aborted fetuses.

MULTIPLE DOSING

Sometimes a parent will miss one or more vaccination appointments and the doctor will say, "That's okay, we'll just give your child three [or four or more] shots today to catch up." Sometimes less advantaged children receive five or more shots in one day (which can equal nine or more organisms if any of the shots are combination vaccines) because it is easier or less expensive for the parents to get them at one time. These are examples of *multiple dosing,* and it is a practice that can cause serious problems for children. It makes sense: The more foreign, disease-causing substances, including chemicals and allergens, you inject into an infant or young child, the more chance there is of adverse reactions occurring. Yet there are those who insist that multiple dosing of vaccines makes good sense.

"It's unfortunate that people believe that [multiple dosing of vaccines harms children]," says Benjamin Schwartz, acting director of epidemiology and surveillance for the Centers for Disease Control and Prevention's National Immunization Program, "because when a new vaccine comes along it provides a wonderful opportunity for us to prevent additional diseases. It would be horrible if some unfounded fears led to underutilization of these important products."

The CDC insists that combining vaccinations saves time and money for parents, and causes less trauma for the child. But are any of these supposed savings worth the price of possibly injuring a child?

At least one government official doesn't think so. Congressman Dan Burton, R-IN, who chaired the US House Committee on Government Reform that has looked at vaccine safety issues, has two grandchildren who had adverse reactions to vaccines. His granddaughter nearly died after receiving a hepatitis B vaccine, and her brother became autistic, he has stated, after being injected with nine different vaccines on the same day.

Concerns About Multiple Dosing

Dr. Marcel Kinsbourne of Tufts University expressed his concerns about multiple dosing to the House Committee on Government Reform when he was asked to speak on the subject of vaccine safety. Dr. Kinsbourne told his audience that "when several vaccines are given at the same time, they may have adverse effects that none of the individual vaccines have when they are given by themselves. Giving many vaccines at the same time is becoming increasingly prevalent, especially to 'captive audiences' like infants. A possible example is measles and mumps vaccines as administered simultaneously in MMR. There is reason to suspect that this combination may cause inflammatory bowel disease and developmental regression into an autistic state in some children in the second year of life."

One significant concern among critics, including myself, who oppose multiple dosing is the fact that researchers are now developing more combination vaccines than those already on the market (such as MMR and DTP/DTaP). One plan was to add the varicella vaccine to MMR (MMRV). This did not prove to be advantageous because the side effects seen after the combination exceeded those seen after the individual vaccines. Another is the design of a super-vaccine, which may contain the genetic material from more than twenty viruses, bacteria, and other disease-causing organisms in one oral form to be given at birth (see chapter 19).

Although the recommended schedule allows up to fourteen vaccines in one day, this is not part of my routine practice. I even suggest that the individual components of the MMR vaccine be taken separately. In addition to the added assault on the immune system when more than one vaccine is given, injecting several vaccines makes it virtually impossible to know which one is responsible for any adverse reactions that may occur. The problem at the time of this writing is that vaccine manufacturer Merck & Company has discontinued single measles, mumps, and rubella vaccines. Merck did say that the manufacture of the single vaccines would resume in 2011.

Multiple Dosing in Adults

The dangers of multiple dosing may extend to adults as well. Mass vaccinations are commonplace among adults in the military, and the case of the Gulf War in 1995 serves as a good example. US soldiers sent to the war received seventeen different vaccines plus an experimental drug. Could this mass assault on the immune system be a reason tens of thousands of these soldiers developed Gulf War syndrome years later? Microbiologist Howard Urnovitz, PhD, believes it was. He says that the vaccines weakened the immune system, making the soldiers much more susceptible to environmental toxins and infections. The symptoms of Gulf War syndrome include chronic joint and muscle pain, rash, headache, fatigue, memory loss, personality changes, diarrhea, sleep disturbances, and an inability to concentrate.

Urnovitz analyzed the blood of many sick Gulf War veterans and found that 50 percent of them had abnormal RNA, which is an indication that chromosomal change has occurred. None of the healthy, nonmilitary controls had these abnormalities. Such changes can result from exposure to viruses, bacteria, or chemical toxins. The specific chromosomes damaged in these veterans have been linked to autoimmune diseases such as rheumatoid arthritis and cancer.

HOT LOTS: FACT OR MYTH?

In 1978 and 1979, eleven infants died within eight days of receiving their DTP vaccine. One specific lot of vaccine, number 64201, made by Wyeth, had been given to nine of the eleven babies. Lot 64201 was a *hot lot*—a term given to a vaccine batch that is toxic or more potent than regular vaccine lots.

It has been impossible to uncover the cause of hot lots because vaccine manufacturers are legally protected against having to reveal the number of doses in any given lot, which can run from tens of thousands to several hundred thousand. Therefore, investigators cannot tell whether a given lot is hot because it is toxic, or because it has a large number of doses and thus the number of adverse effects is greater proportionately. Marcel Kinsbourne, M.D., has observed that no hot lots have ever been withdrawn from the market based on VAERS investigation.

The World Health Organization (WHO), the CDC, and vaccine manufacturers say the idea of hot lots is a misconception. WHO insists "there is little, if any, evidence linking vaccination with permanent health problems or death" and that just because negative reactions are reported to VAERS does not mean the vaccine caused them.

ROTAVIRUS VACCINE: AN "EXPERIMENT" GONE BAD

Rotavirus is the most common cause of diarrhea in infants and young children in the United States. By the time children reach the age of five years, they have probably had at least one rotavirus infection, but the highest number of cases—and the greatest risk—is in children between six and twenty-four months of age. Rotavirus kills about thirty children every year in the US.

In March 1998, the CDC's Advisory Committee on Immunization Practices (ACIP) approved a live rotavirus vaccine made by genetically combining a human rotavirus strain with one from a monkey. FDA approval followed on August 31, 1998. Nearly twenty years of research had led up to these moments. But excitement soon turned to concern and fear. In November 1999, the vaccine was pulled from the market because it was linked with ninety-nine reports of a rare bowel obstruction called intussusception and at least one death in infants. Without proper treatment, which may include surgery, intussusception can be fatal.

Questions Unanswered

Jane Orient, M.D., executive director of the Association of American Physicians and Surgeons (AAPS), questioned why the vaccine was approved in the first place. (See "Conflict of Interest," below, for one opinion.) In a press release, she asked, "What did they [the FDA and CDC] know and when [did] they know it? AAPS has been studying the reports and has concluded that the FDA and CDC may have ignored or concealed data that showed the problems from the outset." She wondered whether the rotavirus incident is just the tip of the iceberg and whether other vaccines have been and are being pushed through without adequate safety testing. She believes that "the tragedy of the rotavirus vaccine might never have happened if the public had access to the data used by the FDA and CDC in recommending the vaccine."

Was this the end of the rotavirus vaccine? No, it was not. A new rotavirus vaccine was approved in 2006 and was recommended for use at two, four, and six months of age. At least 190 cases of intussusceptions in infants receiving the new rotavirus vaccine have now been reported. The CDC has reported that this is not higher than the expected rate of intussusceptions for unvaccinated children.

CONFLICT OF INTEREST

US Representative Dan Burton, R-IN, chairman of the House of Representatives Government Reform Committee during the rotavirus troubles, led an investigation of the members of the two advisory panels that approved the rotavirus vaccine: the CDC's Advisory Committee on Immunization Practices and the FDA's Vaccines and Related Biological Products Advisory Committee. These two entities recommend which vaccines should be placed on the Childhood Immunization Schedule, which is generally adopted by most all of the states.

In addition to the study findings, which indicated there was trouble with the rotavirus vaccine before it got to market, Burton's staff uncovered the following about individuals who voted for the vaccine's approval:

- Some members of both committees owned stock in vaccine manufacturing firms.
- Some members of both committees owned patents for vaccines affected by their decisions.
- Paul Offit, M.D., a member of the CDC advisory committee who voted to add the rotavirus vaccine to the Vaccines for Children program, held a patent on a rotavirus vaccine.
- John Modlin, chairman of the rotavirus working

group of the CDC advisory group, also served on Merck's Immunization Advisory Board and owned $26,000 worth of stock in Merck.

- Three of five members of the FDA's committee who voted for the rotavirus vaccine had conflicts of interest, but they were waived.

Representative Burton concluded that if the conflicts of interest seen on the rotavirus issue are any example of those that exist for other vaccine decisions, "then the entire process has been polluted and the public trust has been violated."

BOTTOM LINE

Are vaccines safe? In 1979, the CDC said: "Vaccinations are recommended and administered to millions of children and other individuals each year on the presumption that the benefits far outweigh the risks. The benefit side of the equation is straightforward: vaccinations can prevent serious disease. The risk side is not as straightforward since it includes factors that are known and others that may exist but have not yet been discovered. It is necessary . . . to maintain surveillance of potential risks of vaccination to continually reevaluate whether individual vaccinations are, on balance, good for people."

So far it appears that the "surveillance" may have been less than adequate. It may be tainted by desires for economic gain by some vaccine manufacturers and for power by some government entities. Individuals who sit on the panels and boards that make the decisions about which vaccines to approve or disapprove may be receiving monetary or other benefits from pharmaceutical companies. Such conflict of interest can make it impossible to get unbiased evaluations of potential vaccines and leaves the door open for insufficient safety tests, ignored adverse reactions, and premature approvals.

That's why it's necessary for you to research both sides of the debate on any vaccine, weigh the information, and consider your child's health and your personal and philosophical feelings about vaccines. Each of the chapters that follow contains information that will help you make the decision that is best for you and your child.

NOTES

Burton, Dan. Statements, see Koch, *CQ Researcher,* p. 654.

Diodati, Catherine J. M. *Immunization: History, Ethics, Law and Health.* Ontario, Canada: Integral Aspects, 1999, 69.

Dynamic Chiropractic Web site: www.chiroweb.com/archives.

Fisher, Barbara Loe. *The Consumer's Guide to Childhood Vaccines.* Vienna, VA: National Vaccine Information Center, 1997.

Halsey, Neal. Testimony of October 1999 before the House Committee on Government Reform, www.house.gov/reform/hearings/health care/99.10.12/halsey.htm.

Incao, Philip. www.garynull.com/Documentsniin/incao_hepatitis_b_vaccination_te.htm.

Katz, Samuel L. Testimony, see Koch, *CQ Researcher,* p. 663.

Kennedy, Ronald. Testimony, see Koch, *CQ Researcher,* p. 651.

Kinsbourne, Marcel. Testimony of August 3, 1999, before the House Committee on Government Reform, at www.whale.com.

Koch, Kathy. "Vaccine Controversies." *CQ Researcher* 10, no. 28 (August 25, 2000): 641–72.

Morbidity and Mortality Weekly Report, March 16, 2007.

National Vaccine Information Center. "Autism and Vaccines: A New

Look at an Old Story." *The Vaccine Reaction* (Spring–Summer 2000).

National Vaccine Information Center Web site: www.nvic.org.

Orient, Jane. Press release of April 6, 2000, at www.aapsonline.org/ aaps/press/nrburton.htm.

Rotavirus information, see www.pcc.com/lists/pedtalk.archive/9909 /0091.html; *Morbidity and Mortality Report,* July 16, 1999, at www .cdc.gov.epo/mmmwr/preview/mmwrhtml/mm4827al.htm; and Michael Devitt, "CDC Pulls the Plug on Rotavirus Vaccine," at www.chiroweb.com/archives17/24/04.html.

Stephenson, Anthony, www.imperial.ac.uk/p8063.htm, August 23, 2006.

Thirteenth World Health Assembly, in Diodati, p. 15.

Urnovitz, Howard. Statements, see Koch, *CQ Researcher,* p. 652.

World Health Organization Web site: www.who.org.

Chapter 3

❈

Mercury in Vaccines: Shots of Danger?

I‌T BEGAN AS AN ATTEMPT TO IDENTIFY THE AMOUNT OF MER-
cury in various foods and drugs. It ended up inciting fear
among parents, concern among researchers, and protests from
manufacturers. *It* was an investigation that led to the realiza-
tion that mercury—a known toxic substance that can cause behavioral problems, learning disorders, and many other medical
conditions—was being injected into infants and young children under the guise of safe, government-sanctioned, routine
vaccinations.

In 1997 Frank Pallone, a congressman from New Jersey, was
concerned about the amount of mercury people might be ingesting in their food and drugs. So he wrote an amendment to
a Food and Drug Administration (FDA) bill in which he asked
the FDA to "compile a list of drugs and foods that contain intentionally introduced mercury compounds and [to] provide a
quantitative and qualitative analysis of the mercury compounds
in the list."

When the bill was signed into law on November 21, 1997 (it

was called the FDA Modernization Act of 1997, or FDAMA), little did anyone know that it would set into motion many years of investigations and accusations, and that people would question the safety and reliability of vaccines and how they are manufactured.

Before we go any farther, I want to say that the situation concerning mercury in vaccines has improved, but we still have a long way to go. There are mercury-free versions of each of the mandated vaccines, and manufacturers have promised to make more available. But there are still mercury-containing vaccines on the market, and many doctors are still using them. The influenza vaccine, recommended for children age six months to eighteen years and for pregnant women, still contains thimerosal as a preservative. Perhaps worst of all, damage has already been done to many children who received dose after dose of vaccines containing ethyl mercury.

This chapter looks at the past, present, and future place of mercury in vaccines. You will learn about the controversy that surrounds the use of mercury, what mercury can do to the body, and what you can do to reduce or eliminate the dangers of mercury for your children and yourself.

MERCURY AND THIMEROSAL

The controversy is over a mercury compound known as thimerosal. Mercury is a metal found in nature in three forms—metallic (or elemental), organic, and inorganic. Everyone is exposed to all three forms of mercury to different degrees. Mercury is in the air as a result of the breakdown of minerals in the earth's surface, and industrial pollution contributes mercury to the air, water, and soil. A significant source of mercury is dental fillings, or amalgams, which can leak varying amounts of mercury into the body depending on the number of fillings in the mouth and their condition.

Mercury has the ability to change from one form to another. For example, metallic mercury can change into methyl mercury, a form that is very common in the environment and one that is a great health concern. Methyl mercury can enter the food supply, particularly seafood.

Thimerosal is a cream-colored powder that is 49.6 percent ethyl mercury by weight. It has been used in vaccines since 1930 as a preservative (it keeps the vaccine from spoiling), and it is effective in fighting off important disease-causing organisms, such as *Pseudomonas aeruginosa* (which causes urinary tract infections and eye infections), *Escherichia coli* (which causes food poisoning), and *Staphylococcus aureus* (which causes food poisoning and various skin disorders). Another disease-fighting preservative, 2-phenoxyethanol, is said to be less effective than thimerosal in keeping these organisms at bay, according to Dr. Stanley Plotkin, author of *Vaccines*.

A 2005 article in the *Los Angeles Times* by Myron Levin stated that Merck's "senior executives were concerned that infants were getting an elevated dose of mercury in vaccinations containing a widely used sterilizing agent." In March 1991, Dr. Maurice R. Hilleman, an internationally renowned vaccinologist, sent a memo to Merck's vaccine division president noting that "6-month-old children who received their shots on schedule would get a dose up to 87 times higher than guidelines for the maximum daily consumption of mercury from fish." The memo continued: "When viewed in this way, the mercury load appears rather large."

This information surfaced at the same time that the number of vaccines given to babies increased and three vaccines—the DTP, Hib, and hepatitis B—were recommended to be given on the same day.

Even though thimerosal contains nearly 50 percent ethyl mercury, it appears few had paid any attention to its potential dangers until Pallone's amendment became law and the FDA was obligated to investigate it. From 1991 to 1999, infants inadvertently received up to 125 times the EPA safe limit of mercury.

HOW THIMEROSAL AFFECTS THE BODY

The amount of literature on thimerosal metabolism and the poisonous effects of ethyl mercury is limited. But toxicologists have assumed that the toxicity of ethyl mercury is the same as that of methyl mercury, another type of mercury about which scientists have some information. Dr. Boyd Haley at the University of Kentucky has shown ethyl mercury to be extremely toxic.

Studies show, for example, that the amount of damage done to the body by methyl mercury depends on the type, level, and duration of exposure to the chemical. To make a comparison, let's look at two items for which the level of mercury is known: a six-ounce can of tuna fish, which contains an average of 17 micrograms (mcg) mercury, and a pediatric dose of hepatitis B vaccine, which contains 12.5 mcg.

So, you might say, what's the big deal? The vaccine contains less mercury than a can of tuna, and many people eat more than one can of tuna during their lifetime.

Here's the big deal. First, how safe is a poison? Mercury is toxic for everyone, including the people who are eating the tuna or who have mercury in the fillings in their mouth (called amalgams; more on mercury fillings below). High levels of mercury can cause brain cells to die, and lower, chronic levels may result in silent or insidious effects that affect the immune system at the cellular level. Thus the first signs of low-level mercury poisoning may be an inability to get rid of the flu, bronchitis, or a yeast infection, or it may lead to cancer. Thus many people may be toxic from mercury and not even know it.

Much more important is the second point: The ethyl mercury in the vaccine is being *injected into the bodies of infants who do not have a fully developed immune system,* and their bodies cannot get rid of the mercury properly. The mercury in the tuna is not injected into the bloodstream; it is eaten, which means it goes through the digestive tract, and the liver has an opportunity to help rid the body of the poison. In infants, the blood–brain barrier, a membrane between circulating blood and the brain that prevents certain harmful substances from reaching the brain, is not yet able to keep out damaging toxins. So mercury sent directly into the bloodstream enters the brain and converts to a form of mercury (inorganic) that remains there, where it does its damage.

Once in the brain, mercury gathers in the areas that affect motor skills and attacks the nerves, affecting emotional and mental functioning. Have you ever heard the term *mad hatters*? In the 1700s, this term was used to describe the people who made felt hats, not because they were crazy about the hats, but because they became "crazy" as a result of making them. Back then, mercury was used to make felt hats, and hatters often developed emotional and behavioral problems, including mental deterioration, timidity, and hallucinations. Is it a coincidence that some of the children who received vaccines that contain ethyl mercury are experiencing these same symptoms? Many experts don't think so.

Researcher G. V. Stajich studied the amount of mercury left in the bloodstreams of pre-term infants in 2000 after they received the hepatitis B vaccine at birth, and found it to be significantly higher than in the blood of the term infant. Another researcher, Michael Pichichero, published a study in 2000 discussing the metabolism of mercury in infants receiving vaccines with thimerosal. It was implied that the ethyl mercury left the bodies of the children shortly following the vaccinations. Dr. Thomas Burbacher clarified this issue in 2005 by doing studies among primates given vaccines with thimerosal. It was found that the ethyl mercury stayed in the blood of the primates only a little more than one week. This was compared with the methyl mercury, which did not leave the blood for at least three weeks. Both forms of mercury traveled to the brain, where the ethyl mercury and methyl mercury became inorganic mercury— which stays a very long time. There was a higher percentage of inorganic mercury from the ethyl mercury than from the methyl mercury (34 versus 7 percent).

What We Know About Mercury/Thimerosal

Experts must look to the studies that have been done on the effects of mercury on the human body to determine the impact of thimerosal. In the late 1950s, women at Minamata Bay, Japan, who ate fish contaminated with methyl mercury gave birth to children with severe neurological and developmental problems. Similar results occurred in Iran, where women ate grain that had been treated with a fungicide containing methyl mercury.

Then there are two studies that looked at the effects of dietary mercury on infants born to mothers who ate large amounts of mercury-containing fish. In a study from the Seychelles, mothers ate fish that contained a high amount of toxin on a daily basis. When the mothers' hair was tested, the results showed high levels of the metal. Yet their infants were not born with developmental defects.

In another study, however, pregnant women in the Faroe Islands also ate highly contaminated fish, but only occasionally. They had high levels of mercury in their hair samples as well. Their children scored low on attention, language skills, and memory. Why did the Faroe Island infants have signs of mercury poisoning while the Seychelles infants did not? Although researchers cannot be certain, some believe it is because the Faroe Island women got their mercury in "bursts"—they did not eat the highly toxic whale meat every day, and therefore their bodies could not adequately handle the toxic shock.

HOW TOXIC IS MERCURY? A CLOSER LOOK

Mercury affects the nervous system and immune system at a very basic level—the cell. It damages the transmission of signals in the brain and in the peripheral nervous system (the nervous system beyond the brain and spinal cord). The damage mercury can do to infants is especially devastating, because:

- The brain is still undergoing rapid development, and mercury can permanently damage brain cells.
- The immune system is not fully developed, which means infants do not have the ability to adequately fight off attacks from foreign invaders, including bacteria, viruses, and environmental toxins.
 The ability to remove toxins, such as mercury, formaldehyde, and aluminum, from the body through the liver has not developed fully.
- In infants, the blood–brain barrier—a membrane between circulating blood and the brain that prevents certain harmful substances from reaching the brain—is not yet able to keep out damaging toxins.

One of the most telling examples of the dangers of this toxic metal is evident in its proposed role in autism. This relationship is explained in chapter 4, where the similarities between mercury poisoning and autism are displayed in a chart. Some experts also believe mercury is a key factor in many neurological and autoimmune disorders, including ALS (Lou Gehrig's disease), Parkinson's disease, Alzheimer's disease, rheumatoid arthritis, chronic fatigue syndrome, multiple sclerosis, and others.

Symptoms of Mercury Poisoning

The above basic facts should make it clear that injecting ethyl mercury into the bloodstream of infants opens the door to problems. And just what kind of problems are we talking about? Some of the most common symptoms of mercury poisoning include:

- Changes in mood and personality, including irritability and shyness
- Loss of sensation
- Vision problems
- Deafness
- Muscle weakness and poor coordination
- Loss of memory
- Tremors

Some experts believe that there is sufficient evidence to show that about 50 percent of the children in the United States who have learning disabilities or mental problems were exposed to prenatal or postnatal toxins such as mercury. (Ways to help prevent exposing your child to mercury are listed in the box at the end of this chapter.)

Ethyl mercury is still found in some vaccines, and there has been reluctance by many manufacturers, government agencies, and health organizations to admit that ethyl mercury is a danger to children's health. And as ethyl mercury is (thankfully) removed from those vaccines in which it still remains, the other issue is: What happens to the countless numbers of children who have been injected with this poison and who have experienced apparent, or not-yet-apparent, medical problems as a result of their exposure?

THIMEROSAL: "NO PROBLEM"

According to a Centers for Disease Control and Prevention (CDC) fact sheet on vaccines, "there is no evidence that children have been harmed by the amount of mercury found in vaccines that contain thimerosal," and "mercury exposure from vaccines containing thimerosal is within the safety margins included in exposure guidelines established by Federal agencies."

However, with the passage of the FDA Modernization Act, the federal government had to take action. On December 14, 1998, the FDA asked manufacturers to provide data on the mercury content of their vaccines. It reissued the request on April 29, 1999, when it required the manufacturers to eventually eliminate or reduce the amount of mercury in their products. (You can see the thimerosal content for some of the licensed vaccines used in the United States at www.immunize.org.)

Yet even though the FDA has ordered manufacturers to do something about mercury in vaccines, it still has had trouble recognizing that thimerosal is a serious health risk. On July 18, 2000, the FDA's William Egan testified before the House Committee on Government Reform, stating that "The risk of emergence of devastating childhood diseases like whooping cough, bacterial meningitis, tetanus, polio, and diphtheria is real. The risk of these devastating childhood diseases from failure to vaccinate far outweighs the minimal, if any, risk of exposure to levels of thimerosal or mercury in vaccines."

The question is, where are the studies that say thimerosal or ethyl mercury in vaccines is safe? At what level is the ethyl mercury in vaccines a health risk?

HOW MUCH IS TOO MUCH?
THE SEARCH FOR TRUTH

In June 1999, after an eighteen-month investigation, the European equivalent of the FDA, the Agency for the Evaluation of Medicinal Products (EMEA), issued its report on the benefits and risks of thimerosal in vaccines. The EMEA stated that "although there is no evidence of harm caused by the level of exposure from vaccines, it would be prudent to promote the general use of vaccines without thimerosal." The Europeans had their say; now it was time for an American investigation.

The Center for Biologics Evaluation and Research (CBER), a division of the FDA, was charged with determining the dangers associated with thimerosal in vaccines. The series of steps CBER took to make this determination is frightening because it brings to mind the question: Why weren't these things taken into consideration before the vaccines were put on the market? Perhaps time will tell on that one.

One of the first things CBER did was look at the standard US immunization schedule and add up how much ethyl mercury children were receiving in vaccines. It found that more than thirty licensed vaccines in the United States contained thimerosal. By the age of six months, any child who got all his or her recommended vaccines had received a great deal of ethyl mercury: 12.5 micrograms in each dose of hepatitis B for a total of 37.5 mcg mercury; 75 mcg from three doses of DTaP; and 75 mcg from three doses of Hib, for a total of 187.5 mcg mercury. The question remained: How much is too much?

Because figures are good only if you have something to compare them with, CBER asked for the federal guidelines for safe levels of mercury intake and hit a hurdle. Thimerosal contains ethyl mercury, and scientists have no toxicity guidelines for this compound. They do, however, have guidelines for its close relative, methyl mercury. Therefore the investigators assumed that methyl mercury and ethyl mercury are equally toxic and asked for the suggested safe levels for methyl mercury from three federal agencies that have this information. Again, they hit a hurdle.

It seems that only two of the three agencies—the FDA, the EPA (Environmental Protection Agency), and the ATSDR (Agency for Toxic Substances and Disease Registry)—agree on the safe limits. It also became apparent that the 187.5 mcg level was not within the safety limits set by the FDA, ATSDR, or the EPA, whose limit is 0.1 microgram of mercury per kilogram of body weight per day. So the 12.5 micrograms of mercury from the hepatitis vaccine injected into, say, an eight-pound (3.6-kilogram) newborn is dramatically higher than the "safe" limit of 0.36 microgram set by the EPA.

The FDA concluded in 2006 that "the exposure to mercury is minimal" because routine infant and flu vaccines total 28 micrograms of ethyl mercury—"significantly below the EPA calculated exposure guidelines for methyl mercury of 65 micrograms during the first six months of life for a child in the fifth percentile of weight." The FDA reasoned that because the baby had been alive for 180 days, it was safe to give 180 days' worth of mercury on one day. The reasoning is faulty. The amount of mercury calculated by the EPA as safe for a five-kilogram infant is 0.5 microgram. If the infant receives 62.5 micrograms, he or she is receiving 125 times the EPA safe level of ethyl mercury. This level actually exceeds the EPA, FDA, ATSDR, and WHO safe levels added together. This is a toxic dose of a very neurotoxic metal.

The flu vaccine, which still contains thimerosal, poses a risk for children and pregnant women. Liquid waste containing more than 200 parts per billion (ppb) of mercury must be deposited at a hazardous waste site. Drinking water cannot exceed 2 ppb mercury. The influenza vaccine contains 50,000 ppb mercury and is recommended for babies and pregnant women.

The Plot Thickens

But there was yet another barrier to understanding the dangers of thimerosal. The study on which the EPA based its guideline involved children who were exposed to methyl mercury daily while still in the womb, as in the cases of the women in the Faroe Island and Seychelles studies mentioned previously. But no one could tell CBER how methyl mercury exposure from the mother before birth compared with exposure in infants who were receiving ethyl mercury injections.

An expert on vaccines, Neal A. Halsey, M.D., director of the Johns Hopkins Institute for Vaccine Safety and a member of the American Academy of Pediatrics (AAP), entered the picture. He was mindful of the growing number of parent advocacy groups questioning vaccine safety that were popping up around the country, and now the uncertainties surrounding CBER's investigations were a new concern. Dr. Halsey and his colleagues at AAP believed doctors should be told about the levels of mercury in vaccines and the possible risks, but officials at the CDC thought that might undermine the vaccination program.

There were many discussions between the AAP and CDC in the days that followed, with much of the talk about delaying administration of vaccines containing mercury during the first six months of life. This meant that the hepatitis B, *Haemophilus influenzae* type B (Hib), polio, and diphtheria-tetanus-pertussis (DTP/DTaP) vaccines would be given after age six months.

This did not happen. The experts believed that delaying any of the vaccines would expose children to the possibility of dangerous infections. But the hepatitis B vaccine was the one most hotly targeted for delay because of its high ethyl mercury content and the fact that it is usually given at birth. Dr. Halsey and other AAP members continued to push for a delay in this vaccine alone. The CDC would not give in, stating that early vaccination with hepatitis B was working: Rates of the disease had decreased dramatically since the vaccination program was started in 1991.

A Compromise

Finally, after a week of negotiations that included input from the AAP, CDC, FDA, and vaccine manufacturers, the two groups reached a compromise. On July 7, 1999, they announced, in essence, that:

- Mothers who are negative for hepatitis B (HbsAg-negative) could postpone the first dose of hepatitis B vaccine from birth until age two to six months.
- Premature infants born to HbsAg-negative mothers could also put off the first dose, and the vaccine should not be given until the infant weighs at least 2.5 kilograms (about 5.5 pounds) and reaches term gestational age.

- Infants born to mothers with hepatitis B (HbsAg-positive) or to those whose status is not known should receive the vaccine at birth.
- In areas where pregnant women are not routinely screened for hepatitis B, all infants should be vaccinated at birth.

After the compromise was reached, Dr. Halsey continued to be concerned about exposing infants to mercury. He noted that researchers need to look beyond the thimerosal in vaccines to accurately determine the amount of mercury infants are exposed to and the effect it may have on their lives. In particular, a mother's fish consumption, her dental history and the presence of amalgams (mercury-containing dental fillings) in her mouth, and whether she took Rho(D) immune globulin (a mercury-containing therapy given to Rh-negative mothers) should also be considered when assessing an infant's exposure to mercury. "No one knows what dose of mercury, if any, from vaccines is safe," says Dr. Halsey. "We can say there is no evidence of harm, but the truth is no one has looked."

The Appearance of Harm

Until more research on ethyl mercury in vaccines is done, scientists must work with the information currently at their disposal. First, we can look at the significant increase in the number of autoimmune and neurological health problems affecting children since 1991, the year the United States added six new vaccines to the required vaccination schedule: live virus polio (five doses); measles, mumps, and rubella (MMR, two doses); Hib (four doses); and hepatitis B (three doses). The government also more strictly enforced the laws that required giving DTP. In 1994, it was announced that one in six of the children in the United States suffered from a neurological deficit.

For example, there is the dramatic increase in the incidence of autism associated with vaccinations—as much as 513 percent in Maryland and more than 300 percent in many other states. The subject of autism is discussed in depth in chapter 4; however, here I want to note that the possible connection between vaccinations and autism was highlighted in the 1980s, when thousands of children had strong symptoms—screaming, shock, seizures, and fever, followed by autistic behavior—after one or more vaccines. Today, autism is more common among children than cancer and cystic fibrosis.

Then there are the great increases in the incidence of autoimmune diseases. Between 1964 and 1980, for example, asthma increased 50 percent in children aged six to eleven years. More than a decade later, the CDC reported that between 1982 and 1992 asthma had increased 52 percent in people aged five to thirty-four years. Other autoimmune diseases have shown an increase in children as well, including diabetes, rheumatoid arthritis, and Crohn's disease. For an in-depth discussion of the relationship between vaccines and autoimmune disease, see chapter 5.

PARTIAL VICTORY: THIMEROSAL-FREE HEPATITIS B VACCINES

At the time this debate was taking place (July 1999), the only two hepatitis B vaccines on the market (Engerix-B from Smith-Kline Beecham—now GlaxoSmithKline—and Recombivax HB from Merck) contained thimerosal. A third hepatitis B vaccine was thimerosal-free, but it also contained Hib vaccine, and this combination is not approved for use in infants younger than six weeks of age.

But as of March 2000, both Merck and GlaxoSmith-Kline had released thimerosal-free hepatitis vaccines. The term *thimerosal-free* is slightly misleading when used to describe any vaccine, because some vaccines that do not use thimerosal as a preservative may contain minute amounts of the substance that gets into the mixture during manufacturing. The Engerix-B vaccine, for example, does contain some thimerosal: It has less than 1 microgram of thimerosal per 0.5-milliliter dose of the vaccine. But this is a 96 percent reduction from the thimerosal-containing product.

Both of the thimerosal-free hepatitis B vaccines are available, and parents who choose to vaccinate their children should ask about them. They are named the same as the mercury-containing varieties.

Why is the arrival of thimerosal-free hepatitis B vaccines a partial victory? Because the immune system of infants less than four months old is not developed enough to handle the assault of not only the ethyl mercury but also the virus, yeast, and aluminum in the vaccine. I do not recommend that any infant whose mother is hepatitis-B-negative receive the hepatitis B vaccine. I think that the unanswered question of a possible link to autoimmune disease is too serious to discount. If the parent wishes to vaccinate with the hepatitis B vaccine, I usually recommend postponing the hepatitis B vaccine (unless the children are at high risk) until after the age of four years.

The assault on the children does not stop with hepatitis B. Not until all vaccines are thimerosal-free; not until all vaccines are adequately tested; not until parents are made fully aware of all their options, and their right to refuse vaccines; not until immunization schedules are allowed to fit the uniqueness of the child rather than the child being made to fit the chart will we begin to truly protect the health of our children.

MERCURY: OTHER SOURCES

As if injecting ethyl mercury into the bodies of infants and children were not bad enough, there are other ways mercury can enter the body and cause harm. One is diet. As the studies noted earlier in this chapter show, pregnant women who eat mercury-contaminated fish pass the mercury along to the fetus. Even after giving birth, breast-feeding mothers who continue to eat fish can pass the mercury to their child through their breast milk.

The use of amalgam, or mercury, dental fillings is another way mercury can pass from mother to fetus and child. Many dentists have abandoned the use of amalgam fillings, but they are still being used by others. Many people still have these old fillings in their mouths. Amalgam is a soft paste that hardens in the mouth after about thirty minutes. Over time, mercury is slowly released from the fillings, unnoticed by people as they chew, brush, and grind their teeth. Some of the mercury escapes as vapor and is breathed into the lungs, while some can be swallowed. Either way, it gets into the bloodstream and circulates through the body. If a woman is pregnant, it can pass through the placenta. The mercury concentrates in the fetus 70 percent higher than it does in the mother. Dental amalgams are a significant source of mercury in breast milk.

The amount of mercury that escapes into the bloodstream depends on how many amalgams a person has and what condition they are in. When you breathe in mercury vapor from the amalgams, 80 percent of it is transported in the bloodstream to the liver, kidneys, and central nervous system, and it attacks the immune system. Once mercury reaches the brain, it is converted to an inorganic form, and some of it may stay for life unless it is removed (see below and chapter 4).

Raymond F. Palmer, PhD, in the Department of Family and Community Medicine at the University of Texas–San Antonio, reported in 2006 that for every thousand pounds of environmentally released mercury, there was a 43 percent increase in the rate of special-education services and a 61 percent increase in the rate of autism in Texas.

Detecting for and Detoxifying Mercury in the Body

In our work with children with autism and other neurological disorders, we use a specific program that identifies mercury and other toxins in the body and then eliminates them. First, we screen hair and blood samples for levels of mercury and other toxic metals. Dr. Amy Holmes published a study in 2003 that looked at the levels of mercury in first-haircut hair in autistic and control children. It was found that there was very little mercury in the hair of autistic children. The control children showed a significant amount. Dr. James Adams had similar findings in a study done in 2008. Florida clinician Dr. Jeff Bradstreet published a study in 2003 showing significant retrieval of mercury in the urine of autistic children after a challenge with 2,3 dimercaptosuccinic acid (DMSA). Very little mercury was recovered in the urine of the control children. Autism, by these studies, was suggested to be a problem with removal of mercury from the body. The children are not able to detox mercury on their own. This will be discussed in the next chapter.

When we treat the children, we use DMSA, and the children release the mercury into the urine. It is rare that we find a child with a developmental problem who does not have increased levels of mercury in the urine after he or she has taken DMSA.

We continue to give doses of DMSA in small amounts over a period of months while we simultaneously add nutrients to the child's diet to replace those that are lost during detoxification. We also periodically test the urine to measure the level of mercury that is being removed and monitor kidney and liver function on a regular schedule. The neurological changes that occur in these children are remarkable and are evident with each dose of the DMSA that we give them. (A more in-depth discussion of the links among mercury, autism, and autism spectrum disorders and the use of detoxification therapy is found in chapter 4.)

How to Protect Your Child from Mercury Poisoning

Here are some steps you can take to protect your child and yourself against the dangers of mercury poisoning.

- At least one brand of every childhood vaccine on the market does not contain thimerosal. When you take your child to the doctor for his or her vaccines, ask for a vaccine that does not contain mercury. Check the package insert yourself to be sure that the vaccine in question is thimerosal-free.
- During pregnancy, avoid having dental work done, or make sure only mercury-free materials are used. The amount of mercury that wears off amalgam fillings is a significant source for a fetus.
- Avoid seafood, especially tuna, swordfish, and shark, during pregnancy or if you are breast-feeding. The fetus is at risk of exposure to methyl mercury during pregnancy when the

mother eats seafood, and infants who are breast-fed can get methyl mercury through breast milk if the mother eats fish.

- If you are pregnant, I'd suggest not getting any vaccines, even the recommended flu vaccine. The mercury can concentrate much higher in the fetus than in the mother, and the fetus cannot eliminate this from its body effectively.

- Drink filtered water. Many municipal water supplies contain mercury. Although the Environmental Protection Agency says that the amount of mercury in drinking water is insignificant and not harmful, some experts worry about the cumulative effects of ingesting mercury every day in water along with all the other mercury exposure.

BOTTOM LINE

At the time of this writing, most thimerosal is out of the recommended vaccines for children. The flu shot, however, still contains significant amounts of thimerosal and it is recommended for six-month-old babies and pregnant women. It is argued that the thimerosal that may be left in some vaccines is "minimal," but if a child genetically cannot detoxify heavy metal, even a very small amount may be too much.

NOTES

Adams, J.B., J. Romdalvik, K.E. Levine, and Lin-Wen Hu. "Mercury in First-Cut Baby Hair of Children with Autism versus Typically-Developing Children." *Toxicological and Environmental Chemistry,* May 2, 2008.

American Academy of Pediatrics Web site: www.aap.org/advocacy/releases/jointvacc.htm.

Bradstreet, J., et al. "A Case-Control Study of Mercury Burden in Children with Autistic Spectrum Disorders." *Journal of American Physicians and Surgeons* 8, no. 3 (2003): 76–79.

Burbacher, T., et al. "Comparison of Blood and Brain Mercury Levels in Infant Monkeys Exposed to Methyl Mercury or Vaccines Containing Thimerosal." *Environmental Health Perspectives* 113, no. 8 (2005): 1015–21.

Centers for Disease Control and Prevention. Joint Statement Concerning Removal of Thimerosal from Vaccines, June 22, 2000, at www.cdc.gov/nip/vacsafe/concerns/thimerosal/joint_statement_00.htm.

———. *Morbidity and Mortality Weekly Report* 49 (2000): 642.

Centers for Disease Control Web site: www.cdc.gov.

Edelson, S. B. "Mercury: The Basic Cause of Major Chronic Diseases of the New Millennium." Unpublished paper.

Environmental Protection Agency. *Mercury Study Report to Congress,* 1997.

Fisher, Barbara Loe. "Shots in the Dark." *The Next City* (Summer 1999): 39ff.

Halsey, Neal A., at www.mercola.com/2000/feb/6/mercury.htm.

HealthWorld Online: www.healthy.net.

Holmes, A., et al. "Reduced Levels of Mercury Burden in First Baby Haircuts of Autistic Children." *Internal Journal of Toxicology* 22, no. 4 (2003): 277–85.

Levine, Myron. " '91 Memo Warned of Mercury in Shots." *Los Angeles Times* (February 8, 2005).

Palmer, R., et al. "Environmental Mercury Release, Special Education Rates and Autism Disorder: An Ecological Study of Texas." *Health Place* 12, no. 2 (2006): 203–9.

Pichichero, M., et al. "Mercury Concentrations and Metabolism in Infants Receiving Vaccines Containing Thimerosal: A Descriptive Study." *Lancet* 360, no. 9347 (2002): 1737–41.

Plotkin, Stanley. Data presented at an August 1999 workshop on thimerosal.

Stajich, G. V., et al. "Iatrogenic Exposure to Mercury After Hepatitis B Vaccination in Preterm Infants." *Journal of Pediatrics* 136, no. 5 (2000): 679–81.

U.S. Food and Drug Administration Web site: www.fda.gov.

Chapter 4

❦

The Autism Debate

In 1943, a child psychiatrist named Leo Kanner described a behavioral disorder in which children are socially withdrawn, exhibit repetitive behaviors, and lack eye contact, meaningful speech, and facial expression. He called the syndrome early infantile autism, which sometimes is still referred to as Kanner's syndrome. Kanner wasn't the first person to use the word *autism*. That honor apparently goes to Eugen Bleuler in 1912, a psychiatrist who used it to describe people who "escape from reality."

At the same time Kanner was documenting his discoveries, another psychiatrist, Hans Asperger, was treating and writing about patients who had nearly the same symptoms, except the children spoke. Today the term *Asperger's syndrome* is often used to describe autistic people who have speech.

Autism (from the Greek word *autos,* meaning "self"), once an uncommon disorder in the United States, has reached epidemic proportions. In the 1960s, the incidence of autism was 1 child out of every 2,000. In the year 2000, it was 1 in 200, and at the time of this writing it has been reported to be as common as 1 in 150.

Why? What is causing this troubling disorder among so many of our children? Is one reason, as many believe, the dramatic increase in the number of vaccines being given to infants and young children? What can we do to stop this epidemic?

This chapter discusses the possible role of vaccinations in autism and other neurological and behavioral disorders. I am not saying that vaccines are the only cause of autism, only that they appear to play a key role in the dramatic increase in the number of cases among vaccinated children. It is interesting to note that autism is not found among the unvaccinated Amish children.

WHAT IS AUTISM AND AUTISM SPECTRUM DISORDER?

When Kanner first described autism, it was thought to be a behavioral disorder only, but research since then has shown it is much more complex. In fact, three parts of the body are involved in autism: the brain, the immune system, and the gastrointestinal tract. This finding led experts to label the condition "autism spectrum disorder." This means that not only do children with autism display a lengthy list of psychiatric disturbances, speech and language problems, sensory abnormalities, cognitive difficulties, and unusual behaviors (all of which are listed and explained in the accompanying chart), but they also have some specific immune system problems and difficulties with their digestive tracts.

If we could peer into the bodies of children with autism, we would see many disruptive processes going on. For example:

- Nearly 85 percent of children with autism have an excess of viruses, yeasts, and other disease-causing organisms in their intestinal tract, which causes them to have diarrhea and problems absorbing nutrients properly. Every day, I see examples of poor nutritional absorption in the autistic children who come to my office. At least 40 percent of my autistic patients have low levels of vitamins A, B_6, and niacin. Eighty percent have abnormal amino acid levels. Most of them have low levels of vitamin B_{12}, magnesium, zinc, and selenium.

- Many of the immune system cells do not behave normally, which results in many autistic children having allergies, asthma, and infections. In the presence of mercury, virus- and yeast-killing cells, called TH1 lymphocytes, are partially replaced by TH2 lymphocytes, which don't have the ability to kill the same organisms as the TH1 cells.

- The liver detoxification system does not function properly, which leaves autistic children unable to detoxify and rid their bodies of heavy metals (such as mercury and aluminum, both of which are found in vaccines), pesticides, or hydrocarbons.

- An increased incidence of seizures and electroencephalogram (EEG, a diagnostic test of brain activity) abnormalities have been seen in autistic children. S. Jill James, PhD, director of the Metabolics Genomics Laboratory at Arkansas Children's Hospital Research Institute, published a study in 2004 describing a methylation defect in many of the families of autistic children. The children struggle to make glutathione, a critical factor in the metal detoxification process in the liver and brain. Diane L. Vargas, M.D., a postdoctoral fellow in the Department of Neuropathology at Johns Hopkins University, demonstrated ongoing inflammation in the brain cells of autistics in 2004. This is what one would see if the child has a genetic methylation defect and cannot make glutathione to detox heavy metal in the liver. Martha Herbert, a pediatric neurologist at Harvard, questioned in a publication in 2006 whether autism is a brain disorder or a disorder that affects the brain. If the child cannot methylate and cannot make adequate glutathione, then the inflammation would affect the brain. It would not be a primary brain disorder, as was originally thought.

These are just a few of the abnormal signs and symptoms experienced by children with autism. But along with the rise in autism, there has also been a similar increase in the number of children with other neurological problems, including attention deficit disorder (ADD), attention deficit hyperactivity disorder (ADHD), dyslexia, and learning disorders. The statistics surrounding these disorders are disturbing. For example:

- About 5 percent of US schoolchildren are estimated to have ADD or ADHD.
- According to the National Institutes of Health, 40 percent of children with ADHD have learning disabilities and 20 to 70 percent of children with ADHD also have conduct disorder (delinquent behaviors). Some experts say that the increase in cases of ADD and ADHD could be associated with better diagnostic techniques, although many others disagree.
- Research published in the *Journal of the American Medical Association* shows that "adults with a history of attention deficit hyperactivity disorder appear to be over represented in the ranks of felons."

Questions about the possible causes of these neurological problems have sent investigators looking in various directions. One of them is into the world of vaccinations.

THE VACCINE–AUTISM CONNECTION

Bernard Rimland, PhD, a psychologist, father of an autistic child, and founder of the Autism Society of America in 1965, established a data bank that includes information on more than thirty thousand cases of autism from around the world. His analysis of the data shows that before the early 1980s, most parents reported that signs of autism were apparent at birth or during the first year of life. But after the mid-1980s, things changed: Suddenly the number of parents reporting that their children developed normally during the first year and a half, and then became autistic, doubled.

What had happened during that time? The combination measles, mumps, rubella vaccine (MMR) was added to the routine child vaccination schedule in 1979 and was given to children at age twelve to fifteen months. At first, the number of children vaccinated was low, but within a few years that changed as federal grants were given to the states so they could provide free MMR vaccines, along with free polio and DTP vaccinations; mandatory vaccination laws were more strictly enforced as well. In 1988, the *Haemophilus influenzae* type B (Hib) vaccine was added to that schedule.

The dramatic increase in autism continued, and so did the number of vaccines and doses added to the childhood vaccination schedule. Between 1993 and 1998, for example, autism increased 513 percent in Maryland. A total of twenty-four other states reported increases of more than 300 percent between 1992 and 1997. And in California, the Department of Developmental Services reported a 273 percent increase in autism between 1987 and 1998. The numbers continue to rise today.

By the end of the 1990s, the average American child was receiving a total of thirty-three doses of ten different vaccines by the time he or she was five or six years old, beginning with a hepatitis B shot at birth and ending with DTP/DTaP and polio vaccinations between four and six years of age. As the number of vaccines given increased, so did the incidence of autism. Not only did the number of vaccines climb but so did the percentage of children receiving them, as federal grants made free vaccinations available to low-income families.

And this fact highlights another interesting observation: Cases of autism were primarily confined to upper- and upper-middle-class families in the 1940s and 1950s. These individuals were the ones who could afford to pay for health care and vaccines for their children, as well as diagnostic testing. As the government made vaccines free to all who could not afford them, autism crossed class lines. Today it is widespread in all socioeconomic groups.

There has been an ongoing discussion in the literature about whether or not to call this an epidemic. Some have said that a change in migratory patterns has brought more autistic children into the United States. Another explanation offered has been that doctors are now diagnosing more cases as autism that carried a different diagnosis in the past. The UC Davis MIND Institute completed a study in 2002 showing that the rise in autism cannot be explained by changes in migration of families and that the epidemic is real.

The parallel increase in vaccinations and autism is only the overall picture. We need to take a closer look at the different factors that could explain it. The least plausible explanation is that we are experiencing a genetic epidemic.

The Mercury/Thimerosal–Autism Connection

Between 1991 and 1999, the United States embarked on what might be labeled a bold, ill-planned experiment: the recommended vaccination of newborns with the hepatitis B vaccine. This vaccine contained 12.5 micrograms of mercury (thimerosal), which is more than twenty-five times the EPA "safe level" of 0.1 microgram per kilogram of body weight per day. This toxic dose was followed by not one but two more doses: one at one to two months and another at six months of age. In addition, infants and children were also given four doses of mercury-containing Hib at two, four, six, and twelve to fifteen months of age; plus four doses of mercury-containing DTP at two, four, six, and twelve to eighteen months of age. By the age of six months, vaccinated children had received 187.5 mcg of mercury—a poison that accumulated in their bodies because production of bile, which helps clear toxins from the body, is not developed in children younger than four to six months.

Ethyl mercury from thimerosal travels to the brain, changes into inorganic mercury, clings to brain tissue, and damages the nervous system. Mercury doesn't go to just any part of the brain; it goes exactly to those areas involved in autism: the cerebellum, amygdala, and hippocampus. The cerebellum is involved in the execution of balance and movement, such as walking and running, and the smooth movements of the eye; the amygdala controls emotional processing; and the hippocampus is involved in the formation, sorting, and storage of memory.

A number of studies have examined the effect of ethyl mercury in the preservative thimerosal on brain tissue and the relation that this may have to autism.

Catherine DeSoto, M.D., in November 2007 published a peer-reviewed study in the *Journal of Child Neurology*, which concluded "that a significant relation does exist between the blood levels of mercury and diagnosis of an autism spectrum disorder."

Leman Yel, of the University of California, Irvine, division of Immunology and Pediatric Allergies, published a study in the *International Journal of Molecular Medicine,* December 2005, showing that thimerosal induces neuronal cell apoptosis or death. In 2003, David S. Baskin, M.D., a Texas neurologist, showed that thimerosal induces DNA breaks, membrane damage, and cell death in cultured human neurons and fibroblasts.

Through all of this, the CDC has maintained that the thimerosal is not a significant risk to children and has not recommended thimerosal-free vaccines over those containing thimerosal. Members of the Academy of Pediatrics have fought at the state level to keep thimerosal vaccines in use. Every year the influenza vaccine is recommended for children and pregnant women without preference to using thimerosal-free brands, but at the time of this writing the flu vaccine still containing thimerosal poses a risk for children and pregnant women.

In 2004, the Institute of Medicine (IOM) also dismissed the risk associated with thimerosal in vaccinations for children. It issued a statement denying a causal link between vaccine thimerosal and autism. The statement was based in part on a study sanctioned by the CDC in 2000. Thomas Verstraeten, a researcher, was commissioned by the CDC to research the effects of thimerosal in vaccines as it related to neurological damage in children. The original study showed a significant risk (at least 7 percent) of developing neurological damage if the child received thimerosal-containing vaccines. The CDC did not authorize the publication of the study in 2000 when the results were divulged. Verstraeten was asked to continue the study in the hope that the risk would be diminished. Verstraeten, in fact, presented an increased risk of neurological damage after thimerosal in the second round of research. The study was reworked another time and was finally published in *Pediatrics,* a very prestigious journal, in 2003 showing no risk of neurological damage after receiving thimerosal. Verstraeten himself said that the thimerosal–autism link needed additional study. No explanation was ever given for the delay of publication and the differences in the outcomes of the various phases of the study. It is appalling to me that the Institute of Medicine used this study to make such an important decision regarding the link between thimerosal and autism.

Since the IOM's 2004 statement, further evidence of a causal link between vaccine thimerosal and autism has mounted steadily. Parents and professionals have questioned the IOM's decision. Several publications have showed a disturbing pattern of a possible link between ethyl mercury and neurological damage in children. Mark and David Geier have published studies from 2005 to 2007 showing a link between heavy metal toxicity—specifically ethyl mercury—on the developing brains of children. Researcher R. Nataf (France) demonstrated abnormal patterns of urinary porphyrins in children in the autism spectrum as an implication of environmental toxicity with heavy metals.

In March 2008, it was announced that the case *Hannah Poling v. United States Department of Health and Human Services* was decided in favor of the plaintiff, and a life care plan was developed to meet the medical needs of the child. This case was decided without having the usual hearing in court and has very definite implications for the vaccine–autism controversy. Hannah Poling has a mitochondrial disorder, which caused her to react poorly when given multiple vaccines containing thimerosal and live viruses. This resulted in fever, regression, and the development of autistic behavior. The vaccines were also thought to have triggered a seizure disorder in the child. Thus the Poling case raises the question: Did she have a mitochondrial disorder genetically, or did the ethyl mercury poisoning cause the problem?

A study published in November 2007 in Portugal reported a significant number of autistic children with mitochondrial disorders. In my own experience, many of the autistic children in my office display signs of mitochondrial dysfunction on physical exam and through blood chemistry. In light of the Poling case and subsequent powerful findings, the American Academy of Pediatrics met with some physicians in the Defeat Autism Now! group through the Autism Research Institute to discuss the best method of treatment for children in the autism spectrum. In fact, even the CDC is willing to admit that the data bank used in the Verstraeten study from 2000 to 2003 may have misled researchers and actually could have resulted in false information about the link between vaccines and autism.

While this seemed to be a breakthrough in the vaccine–autism link, it was announced that three cases in the Vaccine Court in February 2009 were lost by the families of autistic children. Apparently the evidence brought to the court by the families and their attorneys was not convincing enough to prove a link between vaccines and autism. At the same time, several cases were won on their own merits by families of autistic children whose attorneys argued that the encephalopathy suffered following certain vaccines was caused by vaccines. In these cases, the attorneys avoided the term *autism* and presented the encephalopathy as the problem.

It is incredible to me that a controversy still exists over whether or not to inject neurotoxic ethyl mercury into infants and pregnant women—or anyone, for that matter. It is my hope that the IOM's and CDC's overdue acknowledgment of the harmful effects caused by ethyl mercury will come, and soon.

Perhaps there is no way to better illustrate the relationship between mercury and autism than to look at the characteristics of each. The accompanying chart shows the similar and overlapping traits of mercury poisoning and autism in seven categories plus their similar population characteristics. These facts are strong evidence that many of the cases of autism that have been diagnosed in recent years and continue to be diagnosed today are a form of mercury poisoning.

COMPARISON OF CHARACTERISTICS OF AUTISM AND MERCURY POISONING

CHARACTERISTIC	AUTISM	MERCURY POISONING
Movement disorders	Arm flapping, jumping, spinning, rocking, circling; abnormal posture and gait; clumsiness, lack of coordination; difficulties crawling, lying down, sitting, walking; difficulty swallowing or chewing; walking on the toes	Arm flapping, ankle jerks, rocking, circling; lack of coordination, clumsiness; inability to walk, stand, or sit; difficulty swallowing or chewing; walking on the toes
Sensory abnormalities	Oversensitive to sound; abnormal sensation in the mouth, arms, and legs; doesn't like to be touched	Oversensitive to sound; abnormal sensations in the mouth, arms, and legs; doesn't like to be touched
Speech, hearing, language problems	Delayed language or failure to develop speech; mild to severe hearing loss; problems with articulation; word use errors	Loss of speech or failure to develop speech; hearing loss; deafness at very high doses; problems with articulation; word retrieval problems
Cognitive problems	Borderline intelligence, mental retardation: may be recovered; poor concentration, shifting attention; difficulty following multiple commands; difficulty comprehending words; difficulty understanding abstract ideas and symbols	Borderline intelligence, mental retardation: may be reversed; poor concentration and attention; difficulty following complex commands; difficulty comprehending words; difficulty understanding abstract ideas and symbols
Visual problems	Poor eye contact; blurred vision	Poor eye contact; blurred vision

| **Physical problems** | Decreased muscle strength, especially in upper body; incontinence; rash, dermatitis; abnormal sweating, poor circulation, high heart rate; diarrhea, constipation, gas, abdominal discomfort; anorexia, feeding problems; seizures; tendency to have allergies and asthma; family history of autoimmune symptoms, especially rheumatoid arthritis | Decreased muscle strength, especially in upper body; incontinence, salivating; rash, dermatitis; abnormal sweating, poor circulation, high heart rate; diarrhea, constipation, abdominal pain; anorexia, nausea, poor appetite; seizures; sensitive individuals more likely to have allergies, asthma; more likely to have autoimmune symptoms, especially rheumatoid arthritis |
| **Unusual behavior** | Sleeping difficulties; injures self, such as head banging; staring, unprovoked crying, social isolation | Sleeping difficulties; injures self, such as head banging; staring, unprovoked crying, social isolation |

These are just a few of the many similarities between people who have mercury poisoning and those with autism. At the biochemical and cellular levels, there are many additional similarities, which are much too technical to address here. This information was adapted from a heavily referenced research paper, "Autism: A Unique Type of Mercury Poisoning," by Sallie Bernard and associates, copyright © ARC Research, 14 Commerce Drive, Cranford, NJ 07016, April 21, 2000.

The Role of MMR in Autism

One of the vaccines that has been implicated in autism and autism-related disorders is MMR. Before most children even receive the MMR vaccine, they have already been exposed to a total of 187.5 micrograms of mercury through vaccines. All that mercury has many effects on the body, including on the immune system. When mercury attacks the immune cells, it causes decreased activity of the TH1 lymphocytes—a type of white blood cell that fights viruses, parasites, and other disease-causing organisms. Thus the immune system is compromised.

The MMR vaccine—which contains three live viruses—is injected into the bodies of children whose lymphocytes cannot fight off viruses effectively. According to Andrew Wakefield, M.D., a pediatric gastroenterologist in London who has done extensive research on the link between measles vaccine and autism, the measles virus is transported to the gastrointestinal tract, where it multiplies and causes a persistent measles infection. Dr. Wakefield has documented the presence of live measles particles in the gastrointestinal tracts of many autistic children in his practice and believes that the live MMR vaccine may cause children who are genetically at risk to have a chronic measles infection in their intestinal tracts. This infection causes the walls of the intestinal tract to become inflamed, which then expands to the minute openings in the intestinal wall and allows harmful substances from the intestines to cross through the wall into the bloodstream.

Among those harmful substances are morphine-like substances called casomorphin and gluteomorphin, which are introduced from the diet and get carried in the bloodstream to the brain, where they cause abnormal behaviors.

MEASLES VACCINE AND AUTISM: A MISSING LINK?

Andrew Wakefield, M.D., one of the prominent figures in the field of MMR vaccine research, has published several papers on his findings. In an article in the *Lancet* in 1998, he described a group of twelve autistic British children, eight of whom had been developing normally before receiving their MMR vaccinations. These eight children developed autistic behaviors and severe intestinal problems simultaneously (Crohn's disease and other inflammatory bowel diseases) after the shot. Five of these children had had a negative reaction to vaccinations before receiving this MMR dose.

In another study, Dr. Wakefield described twenty-five children who had sudden-onset autism. Twenty-four of the children had traces of measles virus in their bloodstream that matched the genetic makeup of the MMR. Only one of fifteen children without autism had the virus.

In March 1999 at the Second International Autism Conference, Dr. Wakefield explained how children who have a preexisting immune disorder may be predisposed to harboring the measles virus in their intestinal tracts. When these children are given the MMR vaccine, it may stimulate an immune response, which means the body literally attacks its own tissue, and leads to central nervous system damage. He also told of a healthy, normal fourteen-year-old boy who, within one week of receiving an MMR shot, developed strange behavior that was diagnosed as schizophrenia. While receiving an MMR shot at fourteen is not unusual (MMR shots are recommended for adolescents who have not been vaccinated with MMR as infants), developing schizophrenia at fourteen is uncommon, as in males it is usually diagnosed between the ages of eighteen and twenty-five.

BILLY'S STORY

In 1990, at the age of thirteen months, a bright, healthy child named Billy was taken by his mother, Sally, to get his MMR vaccine. Two weeks later, Sally said, things started to change. Before he had received the MMR vaccine, Billy had been alert and sociable. After receiving his MMR, he avoided eye contact, stopped responding to his parents, and lost his language skills.

At age eighteen months, Sally took Billy in for his Hib vaccine, and immediately his behavior got worse. "He started flapping his arms, twirling, and spinning," said Sally, "Noise terrified him . . . He gagged on his food. He exhibited autistic, compulsive and hyperactive behaviors."

Terrified and confused, Billy's parents began taking their son to various professionals who specialized in learning disorders, speech and hearing problems, and psychology. When a pediatrician conducted blood tests and found that Billy had a borderline high titer to rubella, Sally thought this was unusual, given that it had been a year since Billy had gotten the MMR shot. Her research into the medical literature revealed that rubella infection can cause autism in children who have congenital rubella. Therefore, couldn't the live rubella virus in the MMR vaccine do the same thing? Her research convinced her that it could. She also suspected that injecting the live virus into the bloodstream disrupted the immune system and had a negative effect on the immunoglobulin (IgG) levels that aid in the absorption of nutrients in the gastrointestinal system.

Sally sought help from Sudhir Gupta, M.D., PhD, a

professor of medicine and immunology at the University of California. Dr. Gupta started intravenous treatment of immunoglobulin while Sally changed Billy's diet by eliminating casein and gluten products and giving him supplements to help his immune system and gastrointestinal tract. Within weeks, Billy's behavior improved dramatically. His rubella titers dropped and his immunoglobulin levels stabilized. By the age of four, he had regained normal behavior, eye contact, and speech. At age eleven in 2000, he was getting A's in his classes in a regular public school and playing sports. (For more information about the benefits of immunoglobulin treatment in children with autism, see Dr. Sudhir Gupta in the notes to this chapter.)

DTP and Autism

The first indication that the pertussis portion of the DTP vaccine was causing brain inflammation and chronic brain damage arose in the late 1940s, when two separate reports on the phenomenon were published. They were followed in 1955 by research in which the investigator reported that electroencephalograms showed that "mild, but possibly significant, cerebral reactions occur in addition to the reported very severe neurological changes" after DTP shots were given to infants.

Reports of neurological reactions to pertussis continued over the next few decades, but so did administration of the vaccine. In 1981, a study in the journal *Pediatrics* noted that convulsions or collapse and shock resulted from 1 out of every 875 DTP shots given in the United States. Then in 1985, a book that exposed the plight of more than one hundred children who had DTP-vaccine-associated neurological problems was published.

A Shot in the Dark, by Harris Coulter and Barbara Loe Fisher, documented how children who had been developing normally before receiving the DTP vaccine (often given with the polio vaccine) experienced convulsions, high fever, low consciousness, high-pitched screaming, and extreme drowsiness soon after receiving their shot. These children were later diagnosed as autistic, mentally retarded, epileptic, learning disabled, or hyperactive.

This book was instrumental in helping the Institute of Medicine reach its conclusion in 1994 that, yes, DTP did cause brain inflammation and that the inflammation was associated with "a broad range of long-term dysfunction (neurological, behavioral, educational, motor, sensory, and self-care dysfunction)." The National Vaccine Information Center, which was started by Barbara Loe Fisher around the issue of the dangers of DTP and other vaccines, lobbied hard for a safer DTP vaccine. In 1996, the group won that battle when DTaP (a form that contains a portion of, rather than the whole-cell pertussis bacteria) was released to the market (see chapter 7).

The Pertussis–Vitamin A Connection

Another role of pertussis toxin in autism is being explored by developmental pediatrician Mary Megson, M.D., of the Pediatric and Adolescent Ability Center in Richmond, Virginia. She believes that children who have one or both parents who have a genetically inherited condition called G-alpha protein defect (which manifests as night blindness and various parathyroid, thyroid, and pituitary gland conditions) may be at high risk of autism.

According to Dr. Megson, if these genetically predisposed children receive the pertussis toxin in the DTP or DTaP vaccines, which inserts a G-alpha protein defect and depletes the children of their existing supply of vitamin A, they will develop autism. That's because the toxin causes the G-alpha protein to separate from retinoid receptors, which are critical for vision, sensory perception, language processing, and attention. Treating these children with vitamin A results in dramatic improvements in all these areas.

Dr. Megson bases her theory on a study of sixty autistic children who had a family history of G-alpha protein defect. She has seen a dramatic return of speech, eye contact, socialization, and other normal childhood development in these children once they have been treated with vitamin A (cod liver oil) and a substance called Urecholine, which stimulates the hippocampal retinoid receptors. (Remember, the hippocampus is an area of the brain involved in autism.)

Dr. Megson's findings apply to a select group of children who have a specific family history and so provide only one possible cause of autism. However, her research highlights the role vaccines may play in the development of autism.

Autism, Vaccines, and Pregnancy

The possibility that children whose mothers receive live virus vaccines (measles, mumps, rubella, chicken pox) either before, during, or after pregnancy can develop autism is evident in several recent studies. The CDC and vaccine manufacturers have always warned against administering live virus vaccines immediately before, during, and after pregnancy. The Vaccine Information Statement (VIS) issued by the CDC states that "pregnant women should wait to get MMR vaccine until after they have given birth," yet it does not specify how long women should wait. The 1999 *Physicians' Desk Reference* states that "It has been found convenient in many instances to vaccinate rubella-susceptible [at-risk] women in the immediate postpartum period." The VIS also states that "women should not get pregnant for three months after getting MMR vaccine." For the chicken pox vaccination, the warning is to wait until one month after giving birth to receive the vaccination and to not get pregnant for one month after getting the vaccine.

Unfortunately, some doctors and women ignore these warnings, and based on recent studies, the warnings are inadequate. F. Edward Yazbak, M.D., wanted to know if there is a link between administration of the MMR vaccine to women of childbearing age and the development of autism in the resulting children. He collected 240 questionnaires from members of vaccine and parent groups in the United States, the United Kingdom, and Australia and got what he called "unexpected and alarming findings."

Among the 240 responses were twenty-five women (twenty from the United States, four from the United Kingdom, and one from Australia) who had received a live virus vaccine (fourteen received rubella and eleven received MMR) shortly after delivery because their doctors deemed them to be at risk for rubella infection. They were at risk because they had been vaccinated previously for rubella but had failed to develop antibodies. Twenty women gave birth to children who were breast-fed and who developed autism or autism spectrum disorders. Of the remaining five families, three of the children have allergies and one has cerebral palsy.

Dr. Yazbak believes that women who do not develop adequate antibodies to rubella after receiving their initial vaccination during childhood or adolescence may have an immune system condition that leaves them susceptible to rubella. Therefore, revaccinating these women should be avoided, not only because it will not be effective, but because Dr. Yazbak also believes that these women may transmit the tendency to remain rubella-susceptible to their children through breast-feeding. All the children who developed autism did so after receiving their vaccinations (MMR in most cases).

Another subgroup from the 240 consisted of seven women who had received vaccinations during pregnancy—three received rubella, two measles, and one MMR. The seventh mother received hepatitis B during pregnancy and an MMR vaccine five months before she became pregnant. Six of the seven children born to these mothers were diagnosed with autism, and the seventh with autistic spectrum disorder. This last child was one of a pair of twins; the other twin was stillborn.

Subsequent to this study, Dr. Yazbak received twenty-two more reports from women who had received a live virus vaccine either before, during, or immediately after pregnancy. All of them had at least one child who developed autism. Taking all of the reports into consideration, Dr. Yazbak concluded that:

- Giving a live virus to women just before or during pregnancy is inappropriate.
- Postpartum vaccination with MMR or rubella vaccines may not be safe, as there are possible risks to the child through breast milk.

TREATING VACCINE-RELATED AUTISM: ONE APPROACH

In our office, we have seen more than nine thousand children with autism from ten countries since 1996 and several thousand with attention deficit hyperactivity disorder (ADHD). I believe these children have been poisoned by mercury from various sources, including directly through injections of vaccines (hepatitis B, DTP, and Hib) and indirectly through the placenta and breast milk through the mother's diet (fish), amalgam fillings, environmental exposure (for example, water and air pollution), and, for Rh-negative mothers, the use of Rho(D) immune globulin, a product that lessens the chance of a reaction between a mother and her newborn. Thimerosal was removed from one of the major brands of Rho(D) immune globulin in 2002. The product containing thimerosal was not taken out of circulation at that time, however, and many pregnant women received the immune globulin containing thimerosal for years following 2002. Greater than 40 percent of the autistic children in my practice have been born to a mother who had at least one injection of the Rho(D) immune globulin during the gestational period. Many have had more than one injection. In contrast, only about 3 to 4 percent of the children out of the spectrum were born to mothers who had the injections of immune globulin.

Mercury normally leaves the body through the bile (a secretion of the liver) and is deposited in the stool. A fetus and an infant during its first few months of life cannot produce much bile, which means the mercury that enters the body must be stored somewhere. Mercury travels in the blood across and into the brain through the blood–brain barrier, which is not fully developed during the first few months of life. Once mercury reaches the brain, it is extremely toxic to the nervous system and can cause a long list of complications (see the "Comparison of Characteristics of Autism and Mercury Poisoning," page 72).

Before We Begin

The approach we use in my clinic for children who have autism, attention deficit hyperactivity disorder, or other autism spectrum disorders is to first do a complete blood workup to determine each child's biochemical profile. We also conduct blood and urine analyses for toxic metals, stool analyses, food allergy tests, and urine porphyrins, as well as checking the levels of various nutrients and amino acids. If indicated, the children are tested for immune function and viral illnesses. Any child who has amalgams must have them removed before treatment can begin. A pediatric neurologist usually does a full neurological examination before the child comes to us.

From a genetic standpoint, I test for methylation problems, specifically doing a blood test for the MTHFR polymorphism, C677T. If children have a problem in this area of chemistry, they will have trouble getting the toxins out of their bodies on their own.

What we see in most of the autistic children we treat is abnormally low levels of essential amino acids, zinc, magnesium, selenium, vitamins A, B_1, B_3, B_6, and B_{12}, and omega-3 fatty acids; the stool samples contain one or more toxic parasites, bacteria, and yeasts; and the urine has high levels of two factors, casomorphin and gliadimorphin, which are morphine-like substances produced naturally in the body. When these substances cross the blood–brain barrier, they cause bizarre or "spacey" behavior, characteristic of autistic children.

The blood and urine analyses usually show several toxic metals, including mercury, aluminum (both found in vaccines), arsenic, lead, and tin. Many of these children have food and inhalant allergies, and their immune systems are impaired, leaving them ill equipped to fight off bacteria, viruses, and other pathogens. Many of these families display methylation abnormalities.

Treatment

The treatment approach for these children has several facets. One is the use of a detoxifier drug approved by the FDA for the removal of lead in children. Called DMSA (2,3 dimercaptosuc-cinic acid), it also can be used to remove other toxic metals, such as mercury and tin. DMSA attaches itself to toxic metals in the body and "escorts" them out through the urine. Treatment with DMSA takes several months, as it can only be given in small amounts several times a week. To assist with the elimination of the toxins, the children take epsom salt baths. The magnesium and sulfate in the baths help the liver in its detoxification process.

During this process, we also address the child's nutritional needs. Because use of DMSA also removes some nutrients from the body and these children already have abnormally low levels of many essential elements, we supplement them with B vitamins, vitamin A in the form of cod liver oil, and various minerals and amino acids. We also stabilize the amount of beneficial bacteria in their colon, as bacterial diarrhea and other gastrointestinal problems are common in autistic children. Children who have low levels of immunoglobulins (which aid in fighting infections and the absorption of nutrients by the gastrointestinal system) may be given intravenous doses of gamma globulin to improve their nutritional status.

The children are also placed on a diet free of casein (a dairy product) and gluten (a substance found in wheat, oats, barley, and rye). Researchers have shown that high levels of casomor-phin and gluteomorphin in the urine of children with autism contributes to unusual, hyperactive behavior. These high levels exist because the enzyme that normally breaks down caso-morphin and gluteomorphin is inhibited by mercury. Autistic children attach casein and gluten from their diet to morphine-like substances, which then circulate throughout the body. So to prevent the abnormal behaviors caused by these morphine substances, we eliminate casein and gluten from the children's diets.

Another part of our treatment approach is for children to participate in speech therapy, behavior modification, and occupational therapy. These treatments work very well in most children, especially the younger ones, and have allowed many of them to be mainstreamed into the school system. This is a simplified version of our treatment approach. There are many other tests, cultures, and follow-up studies that we do to monitor the progress of our patients.

We also use hyperbaric oxygen therapy, which enhances the blood supply in the brain. Dr. Paul Harch of Gretna, Louisiana, has used hyperbaric oxygen therapy for years with autistic children and has found through scanning that the children form new blood vessels in the brain after as few as ten treatments. We have found that many of the children begin to speak through the use of nutrient repletion, detoxification of metals, and use of hyperbaric oxygen therapy.

Results

So far the results have been exceptional. The biggest improvements come when toxic metals are removed from children's bodies. We have seen nearly complete recovery in many children. What they may have on their side is their superior resiliency—the ability to bounce back and heal from damage to the body and brain.

BOTTOM LINE

Autism is a complex disorder, and so, it appears, are the factors that may cause it. A link between vaccines and autism seems to grow clearer and clearer as the evidence mounts. There is also an apparent association between autism and autoimmune disorders, as the majority of autistic children also have gastrointestinal problems, asthma, allergies, or other autoimmune diseases.

This is not to say that every child who gets any of these vaccines will develop autism or behavioral problems. But parents should be aware that the risk exists.

In 1999, researchers uncovered a strong relationship between a family history of autoimmune disorders (for example, rheumatoid arthritis, lupus, and multiple sclerosis) and autism. They found that subjects who had two or more family members with autoimmune disorders were twice as likely to have autism. This number increased to 5.5 times for those with at least three family members with autoimmune disorders, and to 8.8 times when the child's mother had an autoimmune disease.

Mady Hornig, M.D., Columbia University, published a study in 2004 showing that mice with some autoimmune history in their families would exhibit characteristics of autistic behavior if they were given vaccines with thimerosal. In that same year, the IOM was commissioned to study the link between thimerosal and autism. Using several studies including a Danish study and the Verstraeten study (already mentioned), the group found neither the thimerosal nor the MMR vaccine was related to autism and urged that future autism research be directed away from this topic. Dr. Bernadine Healy, former National Institutes of Health director and member of the IOM, was interviewed by CBS News. She stated that she is not in agreement with the decision to abandon research in this area and added, "The question has not been answered."

In the next chapter, you will learn about another link in the chain: the connection between vaccinations and autoimmune disorders.

NOTES

Baskin, David. *Toxicological Sciences Advance Access* 74, no. 2 (May 28, 2003).

Bernard, Sallie, et al. "Autism: A Unique Type of Mercury Poisoning." Paper published by ARC Research, 14 Commerce Drive, Cranford, NJ 07016, April 21, 2000.

California Social Services Department 1998–2005.

Cave, S. "Autism in Children." *International Journal of Pharmaceutical Compounding* 5, no. 1 (January–February 2001).

———. "The History of Vaccines in the Light of the Autism Epidemic." *Alternative Therapies in Health and Medicine* 14, no. 6 (2008): 54–57.

Cody, C. L., et al. "Nature and Rates of Adverse Reactions Associated with DTP and DT Immunization in Infants and Children." *Pediatrics* 68, no. 5 (November 1981): 650–60.

Comi, A. M., et al. "Familial Clustering of Autoimmune Disorders and Evaluation of Medical Risk Factors in Autism." *Journal of Child Neurology* 14, no. 6 (June 1999): 388–94.

Coulter, H. L., and B. L. Fisher. *A Shot in the Dark*. San Diego: Harcourt Brace Jovanovich, 1985.

DeSoto, Hitlan. *Journal of Child Neurology* (November 2007).

Geier, David, and Mark Geier. "Thimerosal in Childhood Vaccines, Neurodevelopmental Disorders and Heart Disease in the United States." *Journal of American Physicians and Surgeons* 8, no. 1 (Spring 2003): 6–11.

———. "A Meta-Analysis Epidemiological Assessment of Neurodevelopmental Disorders Following Vaccines Administered from 1994 Through 2000 in the United States." *Neuroendocrinology Letters* 27, no. 4 (2006).

———. "A Prospective Study of Mercury Toxicity Biomarkers in Autistic Spectrum Disorders." *Journal of Toxicology and Environmental Health* 70, no. 20 (2007): 1723–30.

Gupta, Sudhir. "Dysregulated Immune System in Children with Autism: Beneficial Effects of Intravenous Immune Globulin on Autistic Characteristics." *Journal of Autism and Developmental Disorders* 26, no. 4 (August 1996): 439–52.

———. "Treatment of Children with Autism with Intravenous Immunoglobulin." *Journal of Child Neurology* 14, no. 3 (March 1999): 203–5.

Hannah Poling Case. The Department of Health and Human Services, March 2008.

Harch, P., and V. McCullough. *The Oxygen Revolution.* Long Island City, New York: Hatherleigh Press, 2007.

Healy, B. CBS News Report, May 2008.

Herbert, M. "Autism: A Brain Disorder or Disorder That Affects Brain?" *Clinical Neuropsychiatry* 2 (2006): 354–79.

Institute of Medicine, Committee on Immunization Safety Review. Vaccines and Autism. "Executive Summary." Washington, DC: National Academics Press, 2004.

James, S. J., et al. "Metabolic Biomarkers of Increased Oxidative Stress and Impaired Methylation Capacity in Children with Autism." *American Journal of Clinical Nutrition* 80 (2004): 1611–17.

———. "Thimerosal Neurotoxicity Is Associated with Glutathione Depletion: Protection with Glutathione Precursors." *Neurotoxicology* 26, no. 1 (2005): 1–8.

Knivsberg, A. M., et al. "Reports on Dietary Intervention in Autistic Disorders." *Nutritional Neuroscience* 4, no. 1 (2001): 25–37.

Megson, M. N. "Is Autism a G-alpha Protein Defect Reversible with Natural Vitamin A?" *Medical Hypotheses* 54, no. 6 (June 2000): 979–83.

Nataf, R., et al. "Porphyrinuria in Childhood Autistic Disorders: Implication for Environmental Toxicity." *Toxicology and Applied Pharmacology* 214, no. 2 (2006): 99–108.

National Vaccine Information Center. "Autism and Vaccines: A New Look at an Old Story." *The Vaccine Reaction* (Spring–Summer 2000).

O'Hara, W. H., and G. M. Szakacs. "The Recovery of a Child with Autism Spectrum Disorder Through Biomedical Interventions." *Alternative Therapies in Health and Medicine* 14, no. 6 (November–December 2008): 42–44.

Oliveria, G., A. Ataide, and C. Marques. "Epidemiology of Autism Spectrum Disorder in Portugal: Prevalence, Clinical Characteristics, and Medical Conditions." *Developmental Medicine and Child Neurology* 49, no. 10 (2007).

Poling, J. S., and R. E. Frye. "Developmental Regression and Mitochondrial Dysfunction in a Child with Autism." *Journal of Child Neurology* 21, no. 2 (2006): 170–72.

Reichelt, K., et al. "Nature and Consequences of Hyperpeptiduria and Bovine Casomorphins Found in Autistic Syndromes." *Developmental Brain Dysfunction* 71 (1994): 71–85.

Vargus, D. L. "Neurological Activation and Neuroinflammation in the Brains of Patients with Autism." *Annals of Neurology* 57, no. 12 (January 2005): 67–80.

Verstraeten, T., et al. "Safety of Thimerosal-Containing Vaccines: A Two-Phase Study of Computerized Health Maintenance Organization Databases." *Pediatrics* 112, no. 5 (November 2003): 1039–46.

Wakefield, A. J., et al. "Ileal-Lymphoid-Nodular Hyperplasia, Non-specific Colitis, and Pervasive Developmental Disorder in Children." *Lancet* 351 (January–June 1998).

Yazbak, F. Edward. "Autism: Is There a Vaccine Connection?" Parts I, II, and III, at www.garynull.com/Documents/autism996.htm.

Yel, Leman. *International Journal of Molecular Medicine* (December 2005).

Chapter 5

❁

When the Body Attacks Itself:
Autoimmune Disorders

In the United States, we entered the new millennium with a dubious distinction: The frequency of autoimmune diseases in children is higher than it has ever been in the history of medicine. Autoimmune diseases are those in which the immune system mistakenly identifies a good, healthy substance as a bad, harmful one. The result is that the body begins to produce antibodies, which then attack joints, muscles, nerves, or specific tissues or cells.

Despite the advances in medicine and medical technology—or perhaps because of them—we are seeing record numbers of cases of autoimmune disorders. This is especially true among children, where there are rising numbers of juvenile rheumatoid arthritis, juvenile diabetes, pediatric asthma, pediatric Crohn's disease (inflammation and ulceration of the bowel), and Guillain-Barré syndrome (progressive muscle weakness).

Behind cancer and heart disease, autoimmune disease is

now the third leading cause of illness in the United States and in many other developed, industrialized nations. What has caused this rise in autoimmune disorders? One theory is that mass vaccination of our children—who now typically receive more than forty-five vaccine doses before they enter school—is changing or damaging their young, developing immune systems. Our children are being injected with foreign, disease-causing substances before their immune systems have matured to a point where they can cope with such invasions. We are also giving children multiple, simultaneous vaccines, which may cause reactions not seen when a single vaccine is given.

This chapter explores an apparent relationship between vaccination and some common diseases, including asthma, juvenile diabetes (type 1 diabetes), gastrointestinal disorders, Guillain-Barré syndrome, rheumatoid arthritis, and sudden infant death syndrome (SIDS). The jury is still out on whether there is a definite cause-and-effect relationship between vaccinations and all of these disorders. But when it comes to your child, I believe you should be on that jury.

VACCINES AND THE
AUTOIMMUNE RESPONSE

When pre-licensing trials are done on vaccines, researchers typically observe the study participants for hours or several days, and only occasionally for a few weeks or longer, to note any adverse reactions to the product. Such abbreviated methods may be appropriate for determining reactions such as injection site swelling or fever, but autoimmune responses may take months, even years, to emerge. Therefore, because these reactions are rarely seen during testing, the vaccines are ruled "safe." This approach brings to mind the words of Walter Spitzer, M.D., professor emeritus of epidemiology at McGill University, who, when commenting on vaccine safety, said, "There is no problem if you do not look."

Looking for Problems

Some experts make it a point to look. When Marcel Kinsbourne, M.D., a pediatric neurologist, spoke to the Committee on Government Reform on August 3, 1999, on the subject of vaccine safety, he noted that virus particles, such as those injected in a measles, mumps, rubella, or chicken pox vaccine, can remain dormant for months or years before they trigger a disease. Even though damage may be occurring to a child's developing nervous system and brain, said Kinsbourne, many of those injuries may not be noticeable until much later, when they manifest as conditions such as developmental language problems, attention disorders, and cerebral palsy.

When a vaccine enters the body, the immune system responds by attacking its various components. Sometimes this reaction includes an attack on a part of the body that chemically resembles a component of the vaccine. The fluid in the joints, for example, may be attacked in individuals who get the rubella vaccine, as this vaccine is known to cause arthritis in some people. This self- (auto-) attack continues and snowballs into an autoimmune response and, depending on the area of the body under attack, an autoimmune disorder such as rheumatoid arthritis, asthma, or diabetes.

The damaging effects of vaccines on the immune system can be long lasting. A study in the *Journal of Infectious Diseases* looked at the long-term effect of the measles vaccine on interferon production. Interferon is a chemical produced by white blood cells that helps make the body resistant to infection. Interferon production is stimulated when the body is invaded by a virus. In the study, one-year-old infants given the measles vaccine had a dramatic decline in alpha-interferon production, which means the immune system was suppressed. This reduction in their immune system's ability to respond optimally to incoming infectious organisms was observed for one year before the study was ended. Some investigators are concerned that long-term suppression of the immune system may make it difficult or impossible for the body to respond normally to disease and thus set the stage for self-destruction.

One Organization Investigates

In 1986, federal legislation commissioned the Institute of Medicine, National Academy of Sciences, to create a Vaccine Safety Committee to review the medical literature for evidence that vaccines can cause injury and death. The committee found eighteen hundred relevant articles, but its screening criteria for establishing a cause-and-effect relationship between a vaccine and reported adverse reactions were very rigid, requiring expensive case-controlled studies to prove the injuries had been caused by a vaccine. Because these costly studies had not been done, the committee announced that for many of the serious health problems reported to be associated with vaccination the evidence was "inadequate to accept or reject a causal relation."

Yet even the committee could not ignore some of the evidence and acknowledged that brain inflammation and several autoimmune disorders could result from vaccines. Those autoimmune disorders include brachial neuritis and Guillain-Barré syndrome, which can occur after tetanus, DT, and live polio vaccines; thrombocytopenia (destruction of blood platelets responsible for blood clotting) after MMR; and acute and chronic arthritis after rubella vaccination.

THE HYGIENE HYPOTHESIS

It's a law of nature: For every action there is a reaction. That principle is behind the argument made by some experts that the response to the decreased number of infectious diseases in childhood, achieved through the use of mass immunization, has been an increase in chronic autoimmune disorders, such as asthma, diabetes, and rheumatoid arthritis, especially among children, who are the largest group being vaccinated.

Interfering with Nature

In 1997, the *Economist* published an article in which the author-scientists noted that interfering with nature—trying to prevent or treat an infectious disease—can lead to undesirable results. One excellent example is antibiotics, which were developed to destroy disease-causing bacteria. The result is we now have more antibiotic-resistant bacteria than we ever had, and diseases are not responding to antibiotic treatment.

The "hygiene hypothesis" states that being exposed to infectious diseases during childhood provides immunity against those diseases and may prevent chronic problems later in life. The article notes that "intervening in infections may have undesirable effects on the hosts—that is, on people—as well as on the pathogens [disease-causing organisms] themselves." One theory explains that the human immune system has evolved over tens of thousands of years to respond to and be strengthened by invading disease-causing organisms. If that natural tendency to fight these organisms is taken away through the use of vaccinations, the immune system may then attack itself—autoimmune disease.

Some researchers, as you will discover below, believe the hygiene hypothesis may explain the relationship between vaccines and the rise in chronic autoimmune disorders. Their studies show evidence that vaccines may be having "undesirable effects" on both people and the disease-causing organisms.

Disrupting the Immune System

In the November 1997 issue of *Science News,* Harvard Medical School immunologist Howard L. Weiner said that immunization disrupts the activity of the immune system. "If a person has a tendency toward a disease at a certain age, a vaccine might . . . make [him or her] more susceptible later, when other challenges come along." An example of this idea is the belief of many experts that giving the varicella (chicken pox) vaccine to children forces the disease to emerge in adolescence or adulthood, when it can cause much more serious complications than it can during childhood (see chapter 11). Dr. Gary Goldman published information about the varicella vaccine in 2006. He is concerned because adults who used to get a boostering effect when their children or grandchildren got the chicken pox will no longer have this occur as long as the vaccine is given to small children. He has reported that shingles cases are predicted to rise by 42 percent among adults under fifty years of age at a cost of $80 million annually.

Do we have proof that vaccines can weaken the immune system? In a study published in *Clinical Pediatrics,* researchers studied the illness patterns of babies before and after vaccination. A total of eighty-two infants were observed for thirty days before vaccination with DTP and thirty days after the shot. (The three days immediately after the vaccination were not included because it is common for children to develop a fever after receiving a vaccine.) Compared with their health before receiving the shot, the babies experienced a significant increase in diarrhea, fever, and cough during the month after vaccination. There was also a positive association of reported past pertussis infections with allergy and asthma in vaccinated children. The association was absent in unvaccinated children.

Researchers have also found that the tetanus vaccine disrupts the immune system in people with HIV by causing a decline in their T cells, a classic sign of immune deficiency. Ten of thirteen patients with HIV who received a tetanus vaccination had a decline in T cells, and the white blood cells in seven of ten HIV-uninfected volunteers became more susceptible to HIV infection after tetanus vaccination because of their immune deficiency.

UC Davis released a study in March 2006 linking thimerosal with immune system dysfunction. It was shown that there was a disruption in the antigen-presenting cells known as dendritic cells in mice. Maureen Drummond, founder of the Network Organization for Vaccine Awareness and Choice, believes this link is significant: "We have traded off communicable disease for chronic degenerative disease." Today many clinicians who treat children support this conclusion.

JUVENILE DIABETES

Juvenile diabetes, more commonly known as insulin-dependent diabetes mellitus (IDDM, or type 1 diabetes), is a disease in which the pancreas does not produce the hormone insulin. Insulin is needed by the body to transport sugar (glucose) into the cells, which is necessary for cell metabolism and, indeed, the very life of cells. People cannot live without insulin.

More than one million Americans have IDDM, which typically is diagnosed in childhood or adolescence. According to the Juvenile Diabetes Foundation, thirty-five children per day are diagnosed with the disease. Each of these children can look forward to an average life expectancy that is fifteen years shorter than people without type 1 diabetes.

Although the exact cause of IDDM is not known, it appears that something causes the body's immune system to attack the pancreas and destroy the insulin-producing beta cells. Once a person's beta cells have been destroyed, he or she needs to take injections of insulin every day to survive. In the search for what can trigger this cell destruction, some experts have found evidence that vaccines may play a role.

Diabetes and Vaccines: Evidence Mounts

Reports of a link between viral infections and IDDM have been circulating for more than two hundred years, ever since scientists first reported cases in which children developed IDDM after they had had mumps infection. With the introduction of the mumps vaccines came reports that they, too, appeared to play a role in the development of the disease. In the 1970s and 1980s, researchers noted that children were developing IDDM after they received mumps vaccination, measles-mumps vaccination, and MMR.

However, the mumps vaccine is not the only candidate for causing diabetes. During the early twentieth century, scientists discovered that pertussis vaccine caused diabetes in mice. Then in 1949, there were reports in the medical literature that some children who had received the pertussis vaccine had lowered blood glucose levels, or hypoglycemia. Hypoglycemia is an indication that the body cannot control its insulin level. In 1979, two German researchers lent support to that finding when they found that 59 out of 149 children in their study who had adverse reactions to the pertussis vaccine developed symptoms of hypoglycemia.

Diabetes and Vaccines: Large Studies

Several large studies conducted in the 1990s have provided convincing evidence that vaccines may be associated with the development of IDDM. Here are a few of them.

- In New Zealand in 1996, researchers saw a 60 percent increase in childhood diabetes cases after the country had a mass hepatitis B vaccination campaign from 1988 to 1991 for infants aged six weeks or older.
- Finland has had vaccination programs for decades, and J. Barthelow Classen, M.D., a former researcher at the National Institutes of Health, has been documenting a vaccine–diabetes connection there. In *Infectious Diseases in Clinical Practice,* he reported that the incidence of diabetes in Finland was stable in children younger than four years of age until the government modified its immunization schedule. In 1974, a total of 130,000 children aged three months to four years received Hib or meningitis vaccine. Then in 1976, the government added a second pertussis strain to its pertussis vaccine. Between 1977 and 1979, the incidence of type 1 diabetes increased 64 percent compared with the period 1970 to 1976. Overall, childhood diabetes rates increased 147 percent in children younger than three years after all the vaccine changes were made. The rates increased another 40

percent in the 1980s in children aged five to nine after MMR and Hib vaccines were introduced.

- At the annual meeting of the American Diabetes Association in San Antonio, Texas, on June 13, 2000, researchers from Italy presented the results of a long-term study of hepatitis B vaccine and insulin-dependent diabetes. In 1991, the Italian government had initiated a mandatory hepatitis B vaccination program for all children at either age three months or twelve years. Children in other age groups were not vaccinated. In the study, the researchers looked at the incidence of childhood diabetes in both vaccinated and unvaccinated children and found that, overall, those who had received the vaccine were 34 percent more likely to develop diabetes than unvaccinated children. In particular, children who were vaccinated at age twelve were more than two and a half times as likely to be diagnosed with diabetes. Based on these findings, the scientists suggested that the hepatitis B vaccine and when it is given "must be reconsidered to reduce the risk associated with it."

The Newest Threat: Pneumococcal Vaccine

In November 1999, Dr. Classen testified before the FDA's Vaccines and Related Biological Products Advisory Committee and warned that the new vaccine for pneumococcal disease (a bacterial disease responsible for a host of ailments ranging in seriousness from ear infections to meningitis—see chapter 13 for more information), called PCV7, would likely cause a large increase in the number of IDDM cases. The new vaccine is similar in structure to the haemophilus (Hib) vaccine, which has been linked to increases in IDDM. Because the pneumococcal vaccine contains seven different vaccines, Dr. Classen believes that it may be seven times more reactive than the Hib vaccine.

To support his claims, Dr. Classen explained the results of his recently published ten-year study in the *British Medical Journal* in which children injected with Hib vaccine were compared with unvaccinated children. After seven years, the rate of diabetes was elevated 26 percent among vaccinated children compared with unvaccinated children. The bottom line is that there were 58 more cases of IDDM per 100,000 immunized children compared with non-immunized children.

Based on these results, and considering the larger population in the United States compared with Finland, Dr. Classen believes the Hib vaccine could be expected to cause four thousand cases of IDDM a year in the United States. Because the pneumococcal vaccine contains seven vaccines, he projected that it could cause twenty-eight thousand cases of IDDM in the United States each year.

Dr. Classen asked the FDA to delay approval of the vaccine until it could be given without the chance of it causing diabetes, but the FDA did not concur with his request. For now, the passage of time will tell whether Dr. Classen's predictions regarding pneumococcal vaccine and diabetes are valid.

JOSHUA'S STORY

At his fifteen-month well-baby checkup, Joshua received his first MMR vaccine. Until then he'd had no health problems except an occasional cold. Three weeks after receiving the shot, he was diagnosed with insulin-dependent diabetes mellitus.

The first week after the vaccination was uneventful.

Joshua's parents had been told their son could experience a rash, fever, or both seven to ten days after the shot. So when he developed a slight fever on day eight, they didn't worry. But then Joshua became excessively thirsty, urinated a great deal, and was lethargic. He had severe vomiting and diarrhea, and his weight dropped from twenty-one to seventeen pounds in less than three weeks. After two days in intensive care, he was diagnosed with insulin-dependent diabetes.

That was in 1988. Today Joshua does well in school, has many friends, and enjoys computer games. But four to five times a day he must test his blood sugar levels, and twice a day he needs insulin shots. He has learned at a tender age that he must be rigorous about his habits and behaviors, because any change in eating or exercising habits can trigger an insulin reaction, including seizures. And he must live with the knowledge that most people with IDDM have a life span that is fifteen or more years shorter than that of people without the disease.

ASTHMA AND ALLERGIES

Asthma is an allergic condition and the number one chronic respiratory disease affecting children in the Western world today. The prevalence of asthma in Western countries has doubled since 1980. Between 1964 and 1980, there was a 50 percent increase in asthma among children aged six to eleven years. A 52 percent increase was seen for persons five to thirty-four years old between 1982 and 1992, and asthma-related deaths increased 42 percent.

People who have asthma experience recurrent attacks of shortness of breath, cough, wheezing, and production of thick mucus. These symptoms are caused by spasms of the airway tubes (called bronchi) and swelling of the mucous lining of the lungs. Asthma attacks can be triggered by an allergic reaction (to grass or dog hair, for example) or by factors such as an infection, exercise, or toxic chemicals. Asthma can lead to respiratory failure and death.

Asthma and allergies can be caused by several different factors working together, including air pollution, smoking, a weakened immune system, food additives, genetically engineered foods, and a poorly functioning gastrointestinal system. Some experts are adding vaccinations to this list, as there is increasing evidence that the vaccines themselves, or the fact that they prevent children from developing natural immunity to a disease, are triggering asthma in children. Here's what the research shows.

ASTHMA AT A GLANCE

According to the American Academy of Allergy and Immunology in the United States:

- Asthma affects nearly five million children younger than eighteen years of age.
- An estimated 1.3 million children younger than five years have asthma.
- Fifty to 80 percent of children with asthma develop symptoms before the age of five.
- Children with asthma miss a lot of school: ten million absences per year.
- Children with asthma account for 2.7 million physi-

cian visits per year and require two hundred thousand hospitalizations.
- The annual cost of treating asthma in children is estimated at $1.9 billion.

Lack of Disease Triggers Asthma

It may sound strange, but some experts believe that not getting specific diseases (that is, receiving vaccines that then prevent children from getting certain contagious diseases during early childhood) may trigger the development of asthma and allergies. In 1996, for example, British and Danish researchers compared two groups of people aged fourteen to twenty-one in West Africa. One group consisted of people who had not been vaccinated against measles and who had recovered from a 1979 measles epidemic (the vaccine was not available at the time of the epidemic). The second group consisted of people who did not have measles as children and who were vaccinated later.

About 26 percent of the vaccinated young adults had allergic conditions compared with only 13 percent of those who had recovered naturally from measles and were not vaccinated. The researchers concluded that having had the measles prevents allergic sensitivity. At the same time, scientists realize that a measles epidemic has risks as well.

But do cases in Africa translate to conditions in the United States and other developed countries? In 1998, investigators looked at cases of asthma and other allergic conditions in children throughout Western Europe, North America, Australia, and New Zealand and found that these countries have higher incidences of asthma than poorer countries in Asia, Africa, and Eastern Europe. One difference between developing countries and industrialized countries is the very high vaccination rate among the latter. Naturally, there are other differences that could have an impact on the rise in asthma cases, such as air pollution and secondhand smoke. However, studies that compare vaccinated with unvaccinated children show dramatic differences in the number of those who get asthma and allergies.

For example, a study in New Zealand published in 1997 concluded that there may be some component of vaccinations for infants that increases the risk of developing asthma. The researchers looked at 1,265 New Zealanders born in 1977. All but twenty-three had received childhood vaccinations, including polio and DTP. None of the 23 nonvaccinated individuals had childhood asthma, while 23.1 percent of the 1,242 who were vaccinated had asthmatic episodes and 30 percent had consultations for other allergy-related conditions.

A study published in the *Journal of Manipulative and Physiological Therapeutics* (March 2000) compared vaccinated with nonvaccinated children and found that those who received DTP or tetanus shots were 50 percent more likely to develop severe allergic reactions, twice as likely to have asthma, and more than 80 percent more likely to have sinusitis (swelling of the lining of the sinuses) than those not vaccinated. The authors concluded that "asthma and other allergic hypersensitivity reactions and related symptoms may be caused, in part, by the delayed effects of DTP or tetanus vaccination."

In a British study published in 1994, the researchers looked at 446 children: 243 who had received the pertussis vaccine and 203 who had not. Among the immunized children, nearly 11 percent had been diagnosed with asthma, compared with less than 2 percent of those who had not received the pertussis vaccine. Anita Kozyrskyj of the University of Manitoba studied the immunization and health records of fourteen thousand children born in Manitoba in 1995. She found that nearly 14 percent of children receiving the DTP vaccine at two months of age developed asthma compared with 5.9 percent of the children whose vaccines were given more than four months after the scheduled day. K. McDonald in 2008 found that the risk of asthma was reduced by half in children whose first dose of DPT was delayed by more than two months from the regular schedule.

Although these studies do not prove conclusively that vaccines play a part in asthma and allergies, the evidence is compelling. Further research may soon uncover the truth behind this relationship.

GASTROINTESTINAL DISORDERS, VACCINES, AND AUTISM

Gastrointestinal (GI) disorders include a wide range of problems that affect the stomach and intestinal tract, which includes the large and small intestines. Crohn's disease and colitis are two of the more common autoimmune GI disorders, and also those that have been linked with vaccines. Gastrointestinal reflux has been documented in infants receiving simultaneous vaccines. Very few infants had reflux until the hepatitis B vaccine was initiated at birth. I saw many infants on medication for reflux following the introduction of that vaccine at birth.

One researcher whose reports of a probable connection between measles vaccine, autism, and bowel disease have caused some controversy is Andrew Wakefield, M.D., of the Royal Free Hospital in London. Wakefield and his colleagues uncovered this connection while they were studying inflammatory bowel disorders in children. They found a group of twelve previously normal children who had suddenly developed both autism and severe intestinal problems. Eight of the children showed this dramatic change soon after receiving their MMR vaccine.

Wakefield and his team hypothesized that assault from a

virus, either naturally or through a vaccine, can cause chronic inflammation of the intestines and damage to the central nervous system of susceptible children. (See more on the connections among autism, MMR, and GI disorders in chapter 4.)

The probability that both autism and bowel disease could be linked with MMR or measles vaccine use created a wave of criticism from the medical community and especially government officials, who were afraid that Wakefield's reports would scare the public into shunning vaccinations. Wakefield explained that he had not proved the relationship, only that it was possible and needed more study. Dr. Wakefield continues his research today. The numbers of children in his studies are greater now, and his results are similar. Andrew Wakefield has been the target of much criticism for making his findings known about the lymphoid nodular hyperplasia (a sign of inflammation) and measles viral particles in the GI tracts of autistic children. He has stood by his findings, and subsequently several researchers in the United States and Japan have duplicated them.

Dr. Wakefield is not the only one who has found a link between autoimmune disorders and autism. A study published in the *Journal of Child Neurology* in 1999 looked at the family medical history of sixty-one autistic patients and forty-six healthy controls. The researchers found that subjects who had two or more family members with an autoimmune disorder were twice as likely to have autism. The likelihood increased to 5.5 times when subjects had at least three family members with an autoimmune disorder and was 8.8 times when the mother of a subject had an autoimmune condition.

VACCINES AND INFLAMMATORY BOWEL DISEASE

In 1995, at the Royal Free Hospital School of Medicine in London, England, researchers believed exposure in measles could be a risk factor for the development of two inflammatory bowel diseases—Crohn's disease and ulcerative colitis. But they wanted to know whether measles vaccination could be a factor as well. So they looked at 3,545 people who had received a live measles vaccine in 1964 and compared them with a control group of 11,407 unvaccinated subjects. The vaccinated subjects were three times more likely to develop Crohn's disease and two and a half times more likely to develop ulcerative colitis than the unvaccinated group.

ARTHRITIS

Scientists know that some viruses, including rubella and influenza, can cause acute arthritis in children and adults. This relationship was given validity in 1991 when the Institute of Medicine (IOM) stated that there is a causal relationship between the rubella vaccine and the development of acute and chronic arthritis. For those affected, severe joint pain usually begins two to three weeks after vaccination (vaccine reaction 9). This acknowledgment by the IOM led the way for individuals who had developed arthritis or arthropathy (a general term for joint disease) to file compensation claims under the National Vaccine Injury Compensation Program (NVICP), which is explained in chapter 22.

An article in *Arthritis and Rheumatology* (1996) reflected on a ruling of the US Court of Federal Claims and the National Childhood Vaccine Injury Compensation Program concerning 124 claims of chronic arthropathy (which included arthritis and arthralgia, painful joints; and fibromyalgia and myalgia, painful muscles) associated with rubella vaccine. Both the NVICP and the court acknowledged the causal relationship that appears to exist between use of the rubella vaccine and chronic arthritis that occurs between one week and six weeks after the vaccine is administered. The court examined the medical records of all the claimants and awarded compensation to fifty-six who met the program's guidelines. Most of these cases involved arthritis and arthralgia.

The rubella vaccine may not be the only vaccine that causes arthritis. In 1998 at the University of Western Ontario in Canada, researchers studied the clinical and genetic background of eleven adults who had acquired rheumatoid arthritis shortly after receiving a hepatitis B vaccination. Nine of the subjects had specific gene characteristics that appear capable of reacting with the vaccine to cause arthritis. The scientists believe that the hepatitis B vaccine, when given to individuals with this genetic trait, may trigger the development of rheumatoid arthritis.

The most debilitating aspect of arthritis is inflammation. C-reactive protein (CRP) is a blood marker for inflammation. M. Pourcyrous published a study in the *Journal of Pediatrics* in August 2007 showing an abnormally elevated CRP in 85 percent of premature infants who received simultaneous vaccines and 70 percent who received one shot at a time.

Colorado physician H. Peter Chase, M.D., found that when infants and young children have a high CRP, they have an increased risk of developing type 1 diabetes in childhood.

GUILLAIN-BARRÉ SYNDROME

Guillain-Barré syndrome is an inflammatory condition in which the immune system starts to destroy the myelin sheath that covers the peripheral nerves. The myelin sheath speeds up the transmission of nerve messages. When this sheath is destroyed, the result is paralysis of the nerves in the legs, arms, lungs, and neck, and often those that control the eyes, heart, and throat.

Guillain-Barré syndrome is neither contagious nor hereditary, and it is rare: 1 to 2 persons per 100,000 get the disease every year. Its cause is unknown, but in about 50 percent of cases it appears after a viral or respiratory tract infection.

In September 1994, the Institute of Medicine released its report "Adverse Events Associated with Childhood Vaccines: Evidence Bearing on Causality," in which it acknowledged a causal relationship between diphtheria and tetanus toxoids and live oral polio vaccine and Guillain-Barré syndrome. The institute's announcement was supported by a few later studies, but overall little research has been done.

- In 1998, a retrospective analysis of Guillain-Barré syndrome in Finland between 1981 and 1986 showed an association between polio virus infection, caused by either the wild (natural) virus or the live vaccine, and an increase in episodes of Guillain-Barré syndrome within a few weeks of a mass polio vaccine campaign. Because there was widespread circulation of wild polio virus immediately before the immunization program began, the researchers cannot definitely prove that the oral polio vaccine was the cause of the increase in Guillain-Barré syndrome cases.
- In Brazil, researchers isolated Sabin-related polio virus vaccine strains from thirty-eight patients with Guillain-Barré syndrome. Nearly all the patients had received their last dose of oral polio vaccine months or years before the onset of the disease.

Guillain-Barré syndrome has been reported following the influenza vaccine, the meningitis vaccine for high school and college students, the human papilloma virus (HPV) vaccine, and others. Gardasil (HPV) vaccine has been associated with at least fifteen cases of Guillain-Barré syndrome when administered simultaneously with Menactra (meningitis vaccine).

SUDDEN INFANT DEATH SYNDROME

Sudden infant death syndrome (SIDS), also known as *crib death,* is a generic term used to classify infant deaths that are unexplained. It is the most common cause of death for children between two weeks and one year of age. The deaths usually occur during sleep and are more likely to occur in the winter than in the summer. Between five thousand and ten thousand cases of SIDS are reported in the United States every year.

Some people, including some medical researchers, believe that vaccines are one cause of SIDS. Harris Coulter and Barbara Loe Fisher, in their book *A Shot in the Dark,* reviewed all available information and medical literature on the topic and estimated that 10 percent of all SIDS cases are caused by DTP vaccine. Viera Scheibner, PhD, author of *Vaccination: 100 Years of Orthodox Research Shows That Vaccines Represent a Medical Assault on the Immune System,* says one study found that in the United States, the peak incidence of SIDS is between the ages of two and four months, when the first two mandatory vaccines are given (at the time of her study, they were DTP and polio), and that another study found a clear pattern of SIDS up to three weeks after immunization. A third study noted that each year, three thousand children die within four days of vaccination. And in the late 1970s, when the Japanese raised their DTP vaccination age from two months to two years, the death claims for DTP in Japan's compensation program dropped.

Yet for the most part, the US medical community refuses to acknowledge the evidence linking vaccines and SIDS. In 1991 and 1994, after reviewing scientific and medical data concerning adverse reactions to various vaccines, the Institute of Medicine published reports that rejected the idea that there was a causal relationship between DTP and DT vaccines and SIDS. However, there was one situation in which the government stepped in and removed a hot lot of vaccine from the market.

On March 9, 1979, the Tennessee Department of Health reported to the Centers for Disease Control that there had been four unexplained infant deaths since November 1978. All the infants died within twenty-four hours of receiving their first DTP vaccination and oral polio vaccine. The deaths were classified as SIDS. But these were not the only SIDS deaths associated with vaccinations in Tennessee. Between August 1977 and March 1978 and then between August 1978 and March 1979, the state reported a total of fifty-two infant deaths from SIDS or unknown causes. An investigation by the US surgeon general led to the withdrawal of lot 64201 of the DTP vaccine.

In the years that followed, several DTP vaccine manufacturers added warnings to their product inserts. In 1984, Wyeth Laboratories stated that "The occurrence of SIDS has been reported following administration of DTP. The significance of these reports is unclear." In 1986, Connaught Laboratories noted that "SIDS has occurred in infants following the administration of DTP. One study has showed no causal connection."

Several other studies considered the issue:

- A study published in the January 1983 issue of *Pediatric Infectious Disease* found a relationship between DTP vaccination and SIDS. The parents of 145 SIDS victims who died between January 1, 1979, and August 23, 1980, in Los Angeles were interviewed about their child's vaccination history. A total of fifty-three children had received a DTP shot; twenty-seven of them had received it within twenty-eight days of their death. Seventeen deaths occurred within one week of the DTP vaccination, and six occurred within twenty-four hours. The researchers stated that these SIDS deaths were "significantly more than expected were there no association between DTP vaccination and SIDS."

- In the April 1986 issue of *Neurology,* researchers reported on their evaluation of the medical records of 103 children who had died of SIDS. More than two-thirds of them had received their DTP vaccination before they died: 6.5 percent died within twelve hours of vaccination, 13 percent within twenty-four hours, 26 percent within three days, and 37, 61, and 70 percent within one, two, and three weeks, respectively.

- In 1987, researcher Alexander Walker published a study in the *American Journal of Public Health* in which he stated that "We found the SIDS mortality rate in the period zero to three days following DTP to be 7.3 times that in the period beginning 30 days after immunization." He also noted that the deaths were associated not only with the first shot but with each additional shot.

- In 1994, two researchers reported in the *American Journal of Epidemiology* that infants die at a rate eight times greater than normal within three days of getting their DTP vaccination.

Dr. Viera Scheibner, who has conducted many studies of SIDS, measured episodes of apnea (breathing cessation) and hypopnea (abnormally shallow breathing) in infants both before and after they received DTP vaccination. The information was gathered using a breathing monitor that generates computer printouts of breathing activity. Dr. Scheibner noted a significant increase in the incidence of both apnea and hypopnea after vaccination and that these episodes continued for several months. Her findings led her to conclude that "vaccination is the single most prevalent and most preventable cause of infant deaths." Her bold statement has caused much debate over the years, and the controversy will continue until researchers can determine the role of vaccines in SIDS.

BOTTOM LINE

Vaccines are supposed to stimulate the body's immune system to produce antibodies to fight off disease-causing organisms, but it appears that in some people they are doing much more. The dramatic increase in the incidence of autoimmune disorders and the parallel increase in the number and potency of vaccinations for infants and young children, along with the fact that many autoimmune disorders are appearing soon after immunizations, are clear signs that there is a relationship among these factors.

It is understandable why vaccine manufacturers disavow any significant cause and effect between their products and autoimmune diseases. Vaccines are big business, and profits are good. And as you will learn in chapter 20, the government insulates manufacturers from liability for vaccine-related injuries. Plus vaccine makers can virtually be assured that their product will get nationwide, if not worldwide, distribution. It's a win–win situation for vaccine makers, but not always necessarily so for the children.

Before your child receives any vaccine, ask yourself the questions provided in chapter 21. In particular, think about whether there is any history of autoimmune disorders in your family. A predisposition to such conditions should be considered when you are deciding whether a specific vaccine should be given to your child. Talk with your doctor. Any tendency toward an autoimmune disease could increase the chance of serious adverse reactions or trigger an autoimmune disease in your child.

NOTES

American Academy of Allergy, Asthma, and Immunology Web site: www.aaaai.org.

American Diabetes Association meeting, San Antonio, Texas, June 13, 2000. At www.msmsmsmsm.com.

Baraff, L. J., et al. "Possible Temporal Association Between Diphtheria-Tetanus Toxoid-Pertussis Vaccination and Sudden Infant Death Syndrome." *Pediatric Infectious Disease* 2, no. 1 (January 1983): 5–11.

Chase, et al. "Elevated C-reactive Protein Levels in the Development of Type I Diabetes." *Diabetes* 53, no. 10 (October 2004): 2569–73.

Classen, J. Barthelow. "Association Between Type 1 Diabetes and Hib Vaccine: Causal Relation Is Likely." *British Medical Journal* 319, no. 7217 (1999): 1133.

Classen Immunotherapies, Inc., press release, November 8, 1999.

Comi, A., et al. "Familial Clustering of Autoimmune Disorders and Evaluation of Medical Risk Factors in Autism." *Journal of Child Neurology* 14, no. 6 (June 1999): 388–94.

Connaught Laboratories, Inc. "Diphtheria and Tetanus Toxoids and Pertussis Vaccine Adsorbed USP." Package insert, July 1986.

Easmon, C. S. F., and J. Jeljaszewicz. *Medical Microbiology. Vol. 2: Immunization Against Bacterial Diseases.* London and New York: Academic Press, 1983, 246.

Economist. "A Virus Hidden in a Vaccine." November 22, 1997.

Ekbom, A., and Andrew J. Wakefield. "Perinatal Measles Infection and Subsequent Crohn's Disease." *Lancet* 344 (August 20, 1994): 508–10.

Fine, J. M., and L. C. Chen. "Confounding in Studies of Adverse Reactions to Vaccines." *American Journal of Epidemiology* 136 (1992): 121–35.

Friedrich, F., et al. "Temporal Association Between the Isolation of Sabin-Related Poliovirus Vaccine Strains and the Guillain-Barré Syndrome." *Review of the Institute of Medical Topics of São Paulo* 38, no. 1 (January–February 1996): 55–58.

Graves, P. M., et al. "Lack of Association Between Early Childhood Immunizations and Beta-cell Autoimmunity." *Diabetes Care* 22, no. 10 (October 1999): 1694–97.

Hovarth, K., et al. "Gastrointestinal Abnormalities in Children with Autistic Disorder." *Journal of Pediatrics* 135, no. 5 (November 1999): 559–63.

Hurwitz, E. L., and H. Morgenstern. "Effects of Diphtheria-Tetanus-Pertussis or Tetanus Vaccination on Allergies and Allergy-Related Respiratory Symptoms Among Children and Adolescents in the United States." *Journal of Manipulative and Physiological Therapeutics* 23, no. 2 (February 2000): 81–90.

Kemp, T., et al. "Is Infant Immunization a Risk Factor for Childhood Asthma or Allergy?" *Epidemiology* 8, no. 6 (November 1997): 678–80.

Kinnunen, E., et al. "National Oral Poliovirus Vaccination Campaign and the Incidence of Guillain-Barré Syndrome." *American Journal of Epidemiology* 147, no. 1 (January 1998): 64–73.

Kroon, F. P., et al. "The Effects of Immunization in Human Immunodeficiency Virus Type 1 Infection." *New England Journal of Medicine* 335, no. 11 (September 1996): 817–18.

McDonald, K., et. al. "Delay in Diphtheria, Pertussis, and Tetanus Vaccination Is Associated with a Reduced Risk of Childhood Asthma." *Journal of Allergy and Clinical Immunology* (2008).

Mitchell, L. A., et al. "Chronic Rubella Vaccine-Associated

Arthropathy." *Archives of Internal Medicine* 153, no. 10 (October 1993): 2268–74.

Montgomery, S. M., et al. "Paramyxovirus Infections in Childhood and Subsequent Inflammatory Bowel Disease." *Gastroenterology* 116, no. 4 (April 1999): 796–803.

Nakayama, T., et al. "Long-Term Regulation of Interferon Production by Lymphocytes from Children Inoculated with Live Measles Virus Vaccine." *Journal of Infectious Diseases* 158, no. 6 (December 1998): 1386–90.

National Vaccine Information Center Web site: www.nvic.org.

Neustaedter, Randall, at www.healthychild.com.

Nussinovitch, M., et al. "Arthritis After Mumps and Measles Vaccination." *Archives of Disease in Childhood* 72, no. 4 (1995): 348–49.

Odent, Michel, et al. "Pertussis Vaccination and Asthma: Is There a Link?" *Journal of the American Medical Association* 272, no. 8 (August 1994): 592–93.

Otten, A., et al. "Mumps, Mumps Vaccination, Islet Cell Antibodies and the First Manifestation of Diabetes Mellitus Type I." *Behring Institute Mitteilungen* 75 (July 1984): 83–88.

Persah, I., et al. "The CHARGE Study: An epidemiological investigation of genetic and environmental factors contributing to autism." *Environmental Health Perspectives* (July 2006).

Pope, J. E., et al. "The Development of Rheumatoid Arthritis After Recombinant Hepatitis B Vaccination." *Journal of Rheumatology* 25, no. 9 (September 1998): 1687–93.

Pourcyrous, M., et al. "Primary Immunization of Premature Infants with Gestational Age <35 Weeks." *Journal of Pediatrics* 51, no. 2 (August 2007): 167–72.

Quast, U., et al. "Vaccine Induced Mumps-Like Diseases." *Developments in Biological Standardization* 43 (1979): 269–72.

Scheibner, Viera. *Vaccination: 100 Years of Orthodox Research Shows That*

Vaccines Represent a Medical Assault on the Immune System. Black-heath, Australia: self-published, 178 Govetts Leap Road, 1993.

Scheibner, Viera, and Leif Karlsson. "Association Between Non-specific Stress Syndrome, DPT Injections, and Cot Death." Second Immunization Conference, Canberra, Australia, May 27–29, 1991.

Stratton, K. R., et al. "Adverse Events Associated with Childhood Vaccines Other than Pertussis and Rubella: Summary of a Report from the Institute of Medicine." *Journal of the American Medical Association* 271, no. 20 (May 1994): 1602–5.

Taranger, J., and B. E. Wiholm. "The Low Number of Reported Adverse Effects After Vaccination Against Measles, Mumps, Rubella." *Lakartidningen* 84, no. 12 (March 1987): 948–50.

Thompson, N. P., et al. "Is Measles Vaccination a Risk Factor for Inflammatory Bowel Disease?" *Lancet* 345 (April 20, 1995): 1071–74.

Tingle, A. J., et al. "Rubella Infection and Diabetes Mellitus." *Lancet* (January 14, 1978): 57–60.

Torch, W. C. "Diphtheria-Pertussis-Tetanus (DPT) Immunization: A Potential Cause of the Sudden Infant Death Syndrome (SIDS)." American Academy of Neurology, 34th Annual Meeting, April 25–May 1, 1982. *Neurology* 32, no. 4, pt. 2; *Neurology* 36, suppl. 1, 148–49.

Walker, A. "Diphtheria-Tetanus-Pertussis Immunization and Sudden Infant Death Syndrome." *American Journal of Public Health* 77, no. 8 (1987): 945–51.

Weibel, R. E., and D. E. Benor. "Chronic Arthropathy and Musculoskeletal Symptoms Associated with Rubella Vaccines. A Review of 124 Claims Submitted to the National Vaccine Injury Compensation Program." *Arthritis and Rheumatism* 39, no. 9 (September 1996): 1529–34.

Weiner, Howard. "The Dark Side of Immunizations." *Science News* (November 22, 1997).

www.winnipegfreepress.com.

Part II

———————— ❁ ————————

THE VACCINES

Chapter 6

❁

Hepatitis B

Every day in the United States, a majority of newborn infants are injected with a vaccine that was created for intravenous drug users, sexually promiscuous men and women, and mothers infected with hepatitis B. None of these infants fall into the first two categories, and less than 1 percent are born to those who fall into the third. Yet the practice of giving hepatitis B vaccine, a compound that often contains toxic substances such as aluminum and allergens like baker's yeast, to infants within hours of their birth continues.

This chapter explores the story of hepatitis and the hepatitis B vaccine. Besides general information about hepatitis B, you will also learn about the controversy surrounding the vaccine: the questionable testing practices, the tens of thousands of adverse reactions associated with the shot, why some experts believe the vaccine should not be given to children, and what you can do to protect your child against possible harm from this vaccine.

A CONTROVERSIAL VACCINE

Of all the vaccines on the market, the one that seems to be the most controversial is hepatitis B, and for several reasons:

- It is the first vaccine most children receive, often on the first day of life.
- It is for a disease very few infants are exposed to unless they are born to mothers who are infected with hepatitis B.
- It is the first genetically engineered vaccine.
- Tens of thousands of adverse effects, some of them very serious, including death, have been reported by parents.
- Up until March 2000, it was one of the vaccines that contained thimerosal (mercury). Now single-dose, non-mercury hepatitis B vaccines are available.

According to the *Morbidity and Mortality Weekly Report, Summary of Notifiable Diseases,* which is published by the Centers for Disease Control and Prevention (CDC), there were only 279 reported cases of hepatitis B in children younger than fourteen years old in the United States in 1996. Only fifty-four of those reported cases occurred in children one year of age or younger. When we consider that there were 3.9 million births in the United States in 1996, the reported incidence of hepatitis B was 0.001 percent for children younger than one year old. Even though these figures reflect reported cases of hepatitis B after the vaccine was in force, the fact remains that less than 1 percent of newborns are at risk for the disease. Yet the recommendation of the CDC, and indeed the standard of care in most hospitals, is to give the hepatitis B vaccine to newborns.

Why does this practice continue? What is the rationale for vaccinating infants whose mothers do not have hepatitis B? Why is the vaccine given to infants when the highest risk period is adulthood? To help answer these questions and look at the controversies surrounding the hepatitis B vaccine, let's first look at some information about hepatitis B and then the vaccine designed to prevent it.

THE DISEASE: HEPATITIS B

Hepatitis B is a contagious disease in which the hepatitis B virus, or HBV, infects and inflames the liver, causing permanent damage in less than 5 percent of those infected. It is not highly contagious, however—you cannot get hepatitis B through casual contact, such as sharing a glass or through sneezing or coughing. The virus is transmitted through exchange of infected body fluids, such as blood or semen. It can enter the body through a cut in the skin, through the exchange of needles used by drug addicts, or through a body cavity, such as the vagina, anus, or mouth. A pregnant woman can pass the disease along to her infant at birth.

How Common Is Hepatitis B?

It is estimated that two to three hundred million people worldwide have chronic hepatitis B. The large range in the numbers reflects the statistics from several different organizations that monitor disease numbers. Regardless of which number you choose, the vast majority of the cases are in Asia and Africa, where the disease affects 20 percent or more of the population. The United States and Canada, however, have typically been among the countries with the lowest rates of the disease, even before the hepatitis B vaccine was introduced in both nations. Today the rate of chronic hepatitis B in both the United

States and Canada is less than 1 percent of the entire population. The CDC notes that "hepatitis B continues to decline in most states primarily because of a decrease in the number of cases among injecting drug users and, to a lesser extent, because of a decline in cases associated with both male homosexual practices and heterosexual practices." If the CDC credits the decline of hepatitis B cases to drug abusers and promiscuous adults, the obvious question concerned parents and doctors must ask is: Why does it continue to recommend vaccinating infants?

Who Is at Risk for Hepatitis B?

Topping the list of people most at risk for getting hepatitis B are intravenous drug users, homosexual men, and prostitutes and other individuals with multiple sexual partners. According to *CDC Prevention Guidelines: A Guide to Action,* these individuals make up 59 percent of all cases of hepatitis B in the United States. Health care workers who handle needles or blood, individuals who live in a household in which someone has hepatitis B, and employees and inmates of correctional institutions also are at risk. Near the bottom of the list are infants born to mothers who have hepatitis B. In rare cases, the disease can be transmitted during an improperly managed surgical procedure. All of these categories together make up between 70 and 75 percent of cases; the other 25 to 30 percent occur in people who say they do not have any of these risk factors.

Not everyone who contracts the virus becomes seriously ill, and not all age groups are affected in the same way. Here are some facts about hepatitis B:

• The younger people are when they first get infected, the less likely they are to develop symptoms soon. Thus, less than 5 percent of infants, 5 to 15 percent of children younger than five, and 33 to 50 percent of people older than five years develop symptoms. However, these same people are more likely to develop a chronic infection: 90 percent of newborns, 25 to 50 percent of children younger than five years, and 6 to 10 percent of people older than five years develop chronic infection.

- Overall, Americans have a 5 percent average lifetime risk of getting infected with hepatitis B, and most of that risk is during adulthood. The age group with the highest reported incidence is twenty to thirty-nine years.

Symptoms and Treatment

Symptoms of hepatitis B can range from none to mild or severe. During the two to four weeks before the liver becomes involved, an individual with hepatitis B may experience loss of appetite, nausea, vomiting, fever, fatigue, and flu-like symptoms. These may be followed by signs that the liver is infected, including dark urine, jaundice (yellow appearance of the skin), fever, pale stools, itching, and a tender, enlarged liver.

Individuals who get hepatitis B can expect one of three things to happen:

- They recover. Nearly 95 percent of all cases of hepatitis B recover completely. Some experience three to four weeks of fatigue, headache, arthritis, jaundice, loss of appetite, tender liver, and nausea; others have no symptoms. People who recover completely from hepatitis B infection have lifelong immunity.
- They develop a chronic infection that eventually, over twenty to forty years, becomes liver cancer or cirrhosis. Hepatitis B is the most common cause of liver cancer.

- They die quickly from an acute infection. This occurs in about two-tenths of 1 percent of all adults who get hepatitis B.

Treatment of hepatitis B includes rest, avoidance of alcohol, and immune system boosters such as interferon. Some people are given hyperimmune globulin, a concentrated form of antibodies specifically for HBV. This treatment is usually given to individuals who know they have been exposed to the virus, such as health care workers who have had contact with the blood of an infected patient.

THE HEPATITIS B VACCINE

When the first hepatitis B vaccine was made in the early 1980s, it was composed of a protein from the plasma (the liquid part of blood) of people who had chronic hepatitis B. But the possibility that other viruses could be passed along with the hepatitis B protein in the vaccine prompted researchers to develop an alternative. Thus researchers developed the first genetically engineered hepatitis vaccine licensed in 1986. This vaccine is also referred to as a recombinant DNA vaccine, meaning that the DNA is altered. The vaccine is made by inserting a portion of the hepatitis B virus gene into a baker's yeast culture, in which this vaccine is produced. (See "Recombinant DNA Vaccines" in chapter 1.)

In 1991, federal immunization officials recommended that hepatitis B vaccine be given to all newborns born in the United States, even though the vast majority of them are in no danger of contracting hepatitis B. This decision was made, said these same experts, because too few of the adults in the high-risk groups were being immunized.

Because the current hepatitis B vaccine does not contain the live virus, it cannot cause the disease it is designed to prevent. However, the vaccine does have a protein that can stimulate the body's immune system in certain ways, some of which appear to cause autoimmune conditions in some people. Bonnie S. Dunbar, PhD, a professor at Baylor College of Medicine in Houston and a pioneer in vaccine research, is one of a growing number of scientists, parents, and health professionals who believe that the hepatitis B vaccine is a serious, perhaps even deadly threat to a portion of the population that may have a genetic makeup that makes them react negatively to the vaccine. Her research suggests Caucasians of Northern European descent may be at higher risk of reacting, but this does not mean the problem does not occur in all groups. In particular, Dr. Dunbar's interest in hepatitis B vaccine intensified after her brother and a research assistant were disabled by reactions to the vaccine.

Researchers at Stony Brook University Medical School, Carolyn Gallagher, PhD, and Melody Goodman, PhD, published a study in 2008 investigating the association between vaccinations with the hepatitis B triple series vaccine prior to 2000 and developmental disability in 1,824 children aged one to nine years. The odds of having to receive special-education services were approximately nine times greater for vaccinated boys (forty-six) as for unvaccinated boys (seven). The findings were statistically significant evidence to suggest that boys in the United States who were vaccinated with the triple series hepatitis B vaccine during the time period in which vaccines were manufactured with thimerosal were more susceptible to developmental disability than were the unvaccinated boys.

How Effective Is It?

According to the CDC, the hepatitis B vaccine is 95 percent effective against hepatitis B disease and infection after a series of three doses is given. Yet one fact that is seldom known by consumers is that researchers, manufacturers, and health organizations are not sure how long the vaccine protects against hepatitis B. According to the *Physicians' Desk Reference,* "The duration of the protective effect" of both the Merck and the GlaxoSmith-Kline hepatitis B vaccines "is unknown at present and the need for booster doses not yet defined." The reason for a lack of immunity as a result of the vaccine is believed to be due to specific characteristics present in the immune system of the nonresponding individuals.

Controversy: Who Should Get the Vaccine?

When it comes to who should get the hepatitis B vaccine, the recommendations of the ACIP (Advisory Committee on Immunization Practices, part of the CDC) differ in one significant way from the list of who is at risk. The ACIP says the vaccine should be given to all children from birth to age nineteen years.

But many experts and consumer advocacy organizations, such as the National Vaccine Information Center, disagree. They note that this age group is at very low risk of the disease, that the disease is not highly contagious, and that given the inadequate testing done in babies and children with different genetic backgrounds before it was licensed, the vaccine should not be mandated and should be used only by high-risk groups. This includes infants who are born to mothers who have hepatitis B. Dr. Dunbar, who has been challenging the federal vaccine policy for years, has been calling for public health officials and government powers to make the vaccine voluntary, especially for newborns. So far her pleas, and those of many other concerned individuals and organizations, have gone unheeded.

There is also the argument by advocates in favor of mandatory hepatitis B vaccination that all infants need to be vaccinated because screening pregnant women for hepatitis B is not being done consistently or adequately by hospitals. In response, those who oppose mass vaccination with hepatitis B vaccine believe it is easier, less expensive, and much safer to screen pregnant women for the disease rather than to subject all infants and children to a vaccine associated with so many adverse event reports.

FEDERAL/STATE GUIDELINES FOR HEPATITIS B DOSING

According to the CDC:

	Infant born to mother infected with HBV	Infant born to mother without HBV	Older child, adolescent, or adult
1st dose	Within 12 hrs of birth	Birth–2 months of age	Anytime
2nd dose	1–2 months of age	1–4 months of age	1–2 months after first dose
3rd dose	6 months of age	6–18 months of age	4–6 months after first dose

The second dose must be given at least one month after the first dose.
The third dose must be given at least two months after the second dose and at least four months after the first.
The third dose should not be given to infants younger than six months of age.

All three doses are needed to get complete and lasting immunity. (However, despite this statement by the CDC in the Vaccine Information Statement, it is not known whether the vaccine is capable of providing complete and lasting immunity according to this schedule.) The shot should be injected into the muscles of the upper arm or thigh.

Who Should Not Get the Vaccine?

The CDC recommends that individuals who fit the following categories should not get the hepatitis B vaccine or should wait:

- People who have had a life-threatening allergic reaction to baker's yeast, which is used to make the vaccine. You can get a blood or skin test to check for this allergy. If anyone in your family has this allergy, you may want to have your child tested before he or she gets the vaccine.
- People who have had a life-threatening allergic reaction to a previous dose of hepatitis B vaccine.
- People who are moderately or severely ill at the time the vaccination is scheduled should postpone the shot until they have recovered. For a different opinion, see "Actions Parents Can Take" in chapter 21.

ROBERT AND RYAN'S STORY

My two patients Robert and Ryan, healthy, lively, identical twins, had both received their MMR, DTP, Hib, and IPV all on the same day. When they were sixteen months of age, their mother, Claudia, told me that the twins had slept for twenty-four hours after receiving the vaccinations and had had a fever when they awoke. Nothing else seemed amiss until, a few days later, Robert's behavior started to change. He began to intentionally injure himself, and tantrums became frequent. His speech, which had been progressing normally before the shots, regressed. Ryan, however, had none of these behaviors. He remained healthy, lively, and outgoing and progressed normally.

When Claudia brought the twins to me, I reviewed their medical history and could find only one difference in their care. While Robert had received his hepatitis B vaccine at one month of age, Ryan had had a cold on the day of the vaccination and did not get his shot until he was five months old. While Robert was plagued with ear infections for months after receiving the hepatitis B shot, Ryan recovered quickly from his cold and had no ear infections. It appeared to me that Robert's immune system had been harmed by the hepatitis B vaccine and that injury could have set the stage for the serious reactions that occurred after the vaccinations at sixteen months.

Today, after months of detoxification at our clinic, Robert has improved significantly, although he is not completely normal.

Side Effects

According to the Vaccine Information Statement (VIS) issued by the CDC, most people who get the hepatitis B vaccine do not experience any side effects. Those that have been reported are as follows:

- Soreness at the injection site, which lasts a day or two: up to one out of eleven children and adolescents and about one out of four adults.

- Mild to moderate fever: up to one out of fourteen children and adolescents and one out of a hundred adults.
- Serious allergic reaction, which can include hives, wheezing, paleness, weakness, fast heartbeat, dizziness, and difficulty breathing: very rare.

The manufacturers of hepatitis B vaccines report that in addition to the adverse effects cited by the CDC, other reactions that can occur in up to 17 percent of people who receive the injection include fatigue, diarrhea, headache, throat and upper respiratory infection, light-headedness, chills, vomiting, stomach pain or cramps, loss of appetite, nausea, sweating, flu, rash, arthritis-like pain, swollen lymph nodes, insomnia, earache, and low blood pressure.

Serious Reactions: An Update

On March 1, 1999, Philip Incao, M.D., testified before the Ohio House of Representatives to explain why vaccination with hepatitis B carries more risks than benefits, with the hope that the state would rethink its practice of mandating the vaccine for all children. He explained that between July 1990 and the end of 1998, a total of 17,497 cases of injuries, hospitalizations, and deaths related to the hepatitis B vaccine had been reported to the Vaccine Adverse Events Reporting System (VAERS). That figure included seventy-three deaths in children younger than fourteen and 146 deaths in people who had received the hepatitis B vaccine alone, without other vaccines.

The most startling figures were seen in the year 1996, when there were 872 reported serious adverse reactions in children younger than fourteen years old: 658 occurred after the children received hepatitis B in combination with other vaccines and 214 happened after receiving hepatitis B alone. Of those 872 children, 48 died: 35 who received hepatitis B vaccine with other vaccines and 13 who got hepatitis B vaccine alone. Dr. Incao compared the total number of hepatitis B cases in 1996 in children younger than fourteen—just 279—with the 872 serious adverse episodes and 48 deaths among children in the same age group who had received the hepatitis B vaccine and concluded that the risks of receiving hepatitis B vaccine far outweigh the advantages. (Dr. Incao failed in his attempt. In August 1999, Ohio mandated hepatitis B vaccine for admission to day care and kindergarten.)

Hepatitis B Vaccine and VAERS

The Vaccine Adverse Events Reporting System has so far received more than sixty thousand reports of adverse effects associated with the hepatitis B vaccine. Many of the reports tell of individuals who have suffered demyelinating- (diseases that damage the myelin—a coating on the nerves—such as multiple sclerosis) and arthritis-like conditions, which VAERS classifies as "unresolved." Assigning this label to these adverse reactions means that the thousands of reports of a possible association between hepatitis B vaccine and sudden infant death syndrome (SIDS), multiple sclerosis, Guillain-Barré syndrome (a paralyzing disease of the nerves), visual disturbances, herpes zoster (shingles), seizures, rheumatoid arthritis, and other medical disorders are never even considered or counted when the CDC and other organizations give statistics on adverse events associated with hepatitis B vaccine. That's because VAERS does not recognize these reactions as being officially associated with the vaccine's use.

Testing and Safety

Many parents would assume that vaccines undergo stringent, long-term testing for safety before they are approved, but in actuality the information that has been made public regarding several vaccines not only has been extremely sparse but also gives rise to questions.

When the FDA allowed the first recombinant DNA hepatitis B vaccine to go on the market in 1986, less than a thousand children were observed for four to five days after receiving their vaccination. In its 1993 product literature insert, Merck stated that "In a group of studies, 1,636 doses of RECOMBIVAX HB [the Merck brand name for the hepatitis B vaccine] were administered to 653 healthy infants and children (up to 10 years of age) who were monitored for 5 days after each dose." (Keep in mind that for hepatitis B vaccine, children on average get three doses.)

If the chance that a certain adverse reaction will occur is 1 in 5,000, how can researchers detect it if they test only 653 children? In addition, reactions to vaccines often take weeks to occur, not five days, and some conditions, such as multiple sclerosis, autism, and learning disorders, may not become fully apparent for months.

The lack of adequate testing of some vaccines has led to what a few experts say is a science experiment, with our children as the guinea pigs.

HEPATITIS B VACCINE TESTS RATED INADEQUATE

When the Institute of Medicine (IOM) published its *Adverse Events Associated with Childhood Vaccines* report in 1994, it made the following observations about the hepatitis B vaccine studies:

- The scientific studies of the hepatitis B vaccine "were not designed to assess serious, rare adverse events; the total number of recipients is too small and the follow-up generally too short to detect rare or delayed serious adverse reactions."
- Neither controlled clinical trials nor controlled observational studies were done to determine whether there was any validity to the thousands of reports that hepatitis B vaccine causes arthritis, SIDS, or demyelinating diseases of the nervous system (those in which there is deterioration of the myelin covering of the nerve cells), such as optic neuritis, multiple sclerosis, and Guillain-Barré syndrome.
- The IOM found that virtually no basic research had been done to identify what caused the adverse reactions and deaths associated with the vaccine. The IOM's report on hepatitis B vaccine and other childhood vaccines concluded that "the lack of adequate data regarding many of the adverse events under study was of major concern . . . the committee encountered many gaps and limitations in knowledge bearing directly or indirectly on the safety of vaccines."

IS HEPATITIS B VACCINE SAFE AND NECESSARY?

YES:

- "Hepatitis B vaccines are among the safest vaccines we have," according to Harold S. Margolis, chief of the Hepatitis Branch at the CDC's National Center for Infectious Diseases, in a statement made to a congressional panel.
- "The hepatitis B vaccine protects children and adults from serious illness and it's a safe vaccine parents can trust," says Acting Health Officer Dr. Maxine Hayes, Department of Health, Washington State.

NO:

- Subcommittee Chairman John L. Mica, R-FL, referred to a study that showed that serious reactions to the hepatitis B vaccine, including eleven deaths, "were sixteen times greater" than cases of the disease itself, a situation he "found shocking."
- Bonnie S. Dunbar, professor of molecular and cell biology at Baylor College of Medicine in Houston and a pioneer in vaccine work, says no. After her brother developed severe multiple sclerosis–like symptoms following a series of hepatitis B shots, she discovered more than 120 articles about adverse reactions to the vaccine. She now crusades against irresponsible use of vaccines.
- Mayer Eisenstein, chairman of the Department of Medicine at St. Mary of Nazareth Hospital in Chicago, says, "The idea of giving this vaccine to a one-day-old baby, a newborn, is preposterous," in a statement made during a 1997 Illinois Board of Health hearing.

SERIOUS REACTIONS:
WHAT TO LOOK FOR, WHAT TO DO

According to the CDC, moderate or severe reactions to hepatitis B vaccine should be reported to and checked by a doctor immediately. If any of these reactions were to occur, they would happen within a few minutes to a few hours after receiving the shot. All adverse reactions should also be reported to the Vaccine Adverse Events Reporting System (VAERS), explained in chapter 22. Signs to look for include:

- High fever
- Behavior changes
- Difficulty breathing
- Hoarseness or wheezing
- Weakness
- Fast heartbeat
- Dizziness
- Hives
- Paleness

More Reasons to Question Hepatitis B Vaccine

As if the sixty thousand adverse effects from hepatitis B reported to VAERS are not bad enough, the FDA admits that VAERS reports represent only 10 percent of the events that have actually occurred. One reason for this frightening statistic is that many doctors don't report deaths or adverse events that happen after a vaccination, because they are too busy. According to a National Vaccine Information Center (NVIC) survey, only 2.5 percent of New York doctors make such reports to VAERS.

Yet parents and others who are told to get a hepatitis B injection are expected to be satisfied with the reassurance by the CDC that "studies show that these side effects are reported no more frequently among those vaccinated than among persons not receiving vaccine." This statement by the CDC is completely unreliable because it is based on only two studies—both of which were conducted more than ten years before the hepatitis B vaccine was being given routinely to infants and children and both of which refer to the old hepatitis B vaccine, not the recombinant-derived vaccine used since 1986. And of course there is a third reason to be skeptical: At least 90 percent of adverse events are not even being reported.

Hepatitis B Vaccine and Other Conditions

The hepatitis B vaccine is being linked with several medical conditions. At the 62nd Annual Meeting of the American College of Rheumatology in San Diego, California, in November 1998, reports from France were that the Ministry of Health had stopped offering hepatitis B immunizations in public schools because the vaccine's use in this age group was linked with newly diagnosed cases of rheumatoid arthritis and was exacerbating other cases that had been in remission. It was also linked with a case of multiple sclerosis (see below).

At another gathering, this time the annual meeting of the American Diabetes Association in San Antonio, Texas, in June 2000, researchers from Italy presented the results of a long-term study of hepatitis B vaccine and insulin-dependent diabetes, noting that children who had received the vaccine were 34 percent more likely to develop diabetes than unvaccinated children (see chapter 5).

Canadian doctors and researchers have also recorded cases of serious problems following vaccination with hepatitis B. Byron Hyde, M.D., chairman of the Nightingale Research Foundation in Ottawa, Canada, has documented hundreds of cases since the early 1990s of nurses and other health care workers who experienced pain, mental dysfunction, fatigue, blindness, skin lesions, measurable loss of IQ, and other difficulties after receiving hepatitis B shots.

Hepatitis B Vaccine and Multiple Sclerosis

There has been some concern in recent years about an association between hepatitis B vaccine and multiple sclerosis (MS), a disease in which there is progressive muscle weakness. Between 1990 and 1999, VAERS received reports of seventy-six individuals who had developed multiple sclerosis or symptoms resembling MS within two to three months after receiving the hepatitis B vaccine. Two separate panels reviewed the information and determined that there was no scientific basis for the claims.

Not everyone agrees with the panels. In France, it used to be customary to vaccinate school-aged children with the hepatitis B vaccine. But in 1998, a French court ruled that SmithKline Beecham's hepatitis B vaccine had caused a child to get multiple sclerosis. As a result of that ruling, the French government halted all hepatitis B vaccination programs in public schools, although the vaccine continues to be used for infants and adults. In addition to this one case of multiple sclerosis, there were reportedly more than six hundred other people who experienced serious immune and neurological problems after their hepatitis B vaccine.

Why Hepatitis B Vaccine Harms: A Theory

Dr. Dunbar and some of her colleagues believe the genetically engineered hepatitis B vaccine causes an autoimmune response. That means the vaccine may trigger the vaccine recipient's body into attacking itself. They suggest this may occur because the vaccine contains substances that are similar to those found in human brain tissues that can cause autoimmune diseases resembling rheumatoid arthritis and multiple sclerosis.

The National Institutes of Health (NIH) has turned down all requests by Dr. Dunbar and her colleagues for grant moneys to study this possibility. The NIH, along with officials of other government agencies, insists that "there is no confirmed scientific evidence that hepatitis B vaccine causes chronic illness, including multiple sclerosis, chronic fatigue syndrome, rheumatoid arthritis, or autoimmune disorders."

"ENCOURAGING" HEPATITIS B VACCINATION

Soon after the CDC recommended that all children receive the hepatitis B vaccine, many states set mandates that require all children to provide proof they have received all three doses of the vaccine before they will be allowed to attend school. Most states require hepatitis B vaccination for individuals entering day care, kindergarten, sixth grade, high school, and college. To see the latest information on how each state has ruled on this issue, as well as types of exemptions individuals can seek to avoid the vaccination, go to www.immune.org.

How States "Encourage" Vaccinations

If you want to encourage people to do something, one of the most effective ways is to offer them an incentive. The CDC has given hundreds of millions of dollars to state health departments in the form of immunization grants since 1965. When the hepatitis B vaccine was added to the recommended list, states could hope to get some of that money if they enforced mandatory vaccinations and tracked them. Today state health officials who cannot provide proof to federal health officials of a certain rate of vaccinations cannot get the funds.

And the amount of funds is substantial. The Comprehensive Childhood Immunization Act of 1993 gave the Department of Health and Human Services (DHHS) the authority to give more than $400 million annually to states that establish a registry that tags and tracks children as they receive their mandatory vaccinations, including hepatitis B vaccine. Each state receives between $50 and $100 per child who is fully vaccinated with all federally recommended vaccines. This tracking system is part of a larger registry program under development by the CDC. (See chapter 20 for information about the registry and more about vaccines and the law.)

Encouragement from Other Sources

Parents are further encouraged to vaccinate their children with the hepatitis B vaccine through the efforts of the nonprofit Immunization Action Coalition, which funds the Hepatitis B Coalition, a national effort to push the vaccine for all children. Funding for this nonprofit comes from private donations, including a grant from GlaxoSmithKline, which manufactures one of the two hepatitis B vaccines on the market. The CDC also gave the nonprofit a $750,000 grant.

BOTTOM LINE

I believe that the controversy and safety concerns surrounding the hepatitis B vaccine make it necessary for all parents as well as adults who may be told to get the hepatitis B vaccine to carefully weigh information from both sides of the issue. In addition to the checklist of precautions provided in chapter 21, consider the following points:

- If you are pregnant, schedule a hepatitis B screening for yourself before your due date to rule out the risk of giving hepatitis B to your infant.
- If you do not have hepatitis B, I do not recommend giving the hepatitis B vaccine to infants. If your decision is to give it with a full knowledge of the possible risks, you can have it given to your child. If the child will go to child care, consult with your child's pediatrician about waiting until just before your child starts day care for the first shot to be given.
- Familiarize yourself with the vaccine exemption laws in your state (see chapter 21). Do not be pressured or intimidated by medical professionals or the hospital into giving your child the vaccine at birth.
- Because yeast is used to manufacture hepatitis B vaccine, people who are allergic to yeast should not get the shot. Your child can be checked for this allergy.

NOTES

Advisory Committee on Immunization Practices. 1999 update. "Hepatitis B Virus Infection: A Comprehensive Immunization Strategy to Eliminate Transmission in the United States."

Centers for Disease Control and Prevention. *CDC Prevention Guidelines: A Guide to Action.*

———. *Morbidity and Mortality Weekly Report.* Summary of Notifiable Diseases, United States, 1996.

———. *Vaccine Information Statements.* May 4, 2000.

Eisenstein, Mayer. Cited in Koch, *CQ Researcher,* 646.

Fisher, Barbara Loe. *The Consumer's Guide to Childhood Vaccines.* Vienna, VA: National Vaccine Information Center, 1997.

———. "Shots in the Dark." *The Next City* (summer 1999): 39, 45.

Gallagher, C., and M. Goodman. "Hepatitis B Triple Series Vaccine and Developmental Disability in US Children Aged 1–9 Years." Graduate Program in Public Health; Stoney Brook University Medical Center; Health Sciences Center, New York. *Toxicological and Environmental Chemistry* 90, no. 5 (September 2008): 997–1008.

Hayes, Maxine. Cited at http://hepatitis-central.com/hcv/vaccines/heph.html.

Hepatitis Information Network Web site: www.hepnet.com/hepb/news012599.html.

Immunization Action Coalition. *Needle Tips and the Hepatitis B Coalition News* 10, no. 1 (Spring–Summer 2008).

Incao, Philip. Testimony in Ohio, March 1, 1999. At www.garynull.com/Documents/niin/incao_hepatitis_b_vaccination_te.htm.

Institute of Medicine. *Adverse Effects Associated with Childhood Vaccines: Evidence Bearing on Causality.* Washington, DC: National Academy Press, 1994.

Koch, Kathy. "Vaccine Controversies." *CQ Researcher* (August 2000): 649.

Margolis, Harold S. Cited at www.biospace.com/articles/111199_pr8int.cfm.

National Vaccine Information Center. "Hepatitis B Vaccine: The Untold Story." *The Vaccine Reaction* (September 1998).

National Vaccine Information Center Web site: www.nvic.org.

Physicians' Desk Reference. Oradell, NJ: Medical Economics, 2000.

Pozzilli, P., et al. "Hepatitis B Vaccine Associated with an Increased Type I Diabetes in Italy." Presented at the Annual Meeting of the American Diabetes Association, San Antonio, Texas, June 13, 2000.

Chapter 7

❃

DTP/DTaP: Diphtheria, Tetanus, Pertussis

THE NATURAL INSTINCT OF MOTHERS TO PROTECT THEIR young is a powerful force in nature. In the late 1970s and early 1980s, such a force was evident as mothers whose children appeared to have been harmed by the DTP (diphtheria, tetanus, pertussis, or whooping cough) vaccine banded together. They fought for the lives of their children and for the lives of those yet to be born. They realized that vaccines against these three diseases could be essential for children's health, but they also knew that their children—all children—deserve safe vaccines, and that DTP was not one of them.

So they founded a nonprofit, educational organization known today as the National Vaccine Information Center. Barbara Loe Fisher, whose own son, Chris, was diagnosed with multiple learning disabilities and attention deficit disorder after suffering a convulsion, shock, and loss of consciousness within hours of his fourth DTP dose and oral polio vaccine in 1980, joined with other parents and lobbied for a safer DTP vaccine. It was a battle they finally won—to a degree—yet the fight for safer, more effective vaccines is not over. The story of what these parents fought for and against, and how it affects you and your children, is in this chapter.

INTRODUCING THE TRIO

Diphtheria, tetanus, and pertussis—these diseases may seem foreign to young parents today, but they can still strike fear into the hearts of grandparents. That's because during the nineteenth century and the early part of the twentieth, diphtheria and pertussis each infected more than a hundred thousand people a year—mostly children—and tens of thousands died each year. Tetanus, although less common, killed several hundred people per year during the same time period.

These terrifying figures prompted scientists to develop vaccines for these child killers. First on the market was a vaccine for pertussis in 1906, followed by a diphtheria vaccine in the 1920s and a tetanus vaccine in 1933. A combined vaccine—DTP—became available in 1946. Although this trio of vaccines was viewed as a lifesaver, it also caused some serious problems. This chapter takes a look at the three diseases DTP was designed to eliminate and the long, bumpy road the vaccine has taken to get to where it is today: still at the center of controversy.

DIPHTHERIA

Diphtheria is caused by *Corynebacterium diphtheriae*, bacteria found in the mouth, nose, and throat of infected individuals.

Healthy people can carry the disease and spread it to others by sneezing, talking, or coughing.

Diphtheria is unique in that the bacteria themselves are actually attacked by a bacteriophage (similar to a virus), which prompts the bacteria to produce a poison. This poison can enter the cells surrounding the infected area, say the throat, and kill them. The buildup of dead cells along with the inflammation caused by the bacteria can cause the throat to become blocked, making it difficult or impossible to breathe.

The poison may also enter the bloodstream and travel to other parts of the body, damaging various organs and the nervous system. Damage to the heart is common and is usually irreversible. If the breathing muscles are affected, pneumonia and respiratory failure can develop.

Symptoms and Treatment

Symptoms of diphtheria include hoarseness, cough, noisy breathing, sore throat, slight fever, irritability, chills, and an increasing inability to breathe. These symptoms are similar to those of croup, another childhood disease. Unless diphtheria is treated early in the disease course, it can be fatal. Between 5 and 10 percent of patients who have diphtheria die. Treatment consists of a diphtheria antitoxin, antibiotics, tracheotomy (opening up the windpipe to allow breathing), and oxygen therapy.

Who Is at Risk for Diphtheria?

Diphtheria most often affects children between the ages of two and five years. In the 1920s, when data were first gathered on diphtheria, about 150,000 people per year had the disease, and 13,000 died annually. The disease peaked in 1921 (206,939 cases), but after introduction of the vaccine several years later, the numbers began to drop. Between 1970 and 1979, there were about 196 cases per year; there were only 4 cases in 1992, with 1 death. Today only 1 case is reported annually in the United States.

The CDC claims that as many as 50 percent of people age sixty and older may be susceptible to diphtheria because they have not had their booster shots. The general recommendation is for everyone age ten years and older to get a Td or TdaP (small *d* because the diphtheria portion of the vaccine is less potent than in the DTP vaccine) booster every ten years.

TETANUS

Tetanus is a painful, often deadly disease that is caused by bacteria (*Clostridium tetani*) that live in soil, manure, and the digestive systems of animals and people. The disease is also known as lockjaw, so named because one of the main symptoms is that the muscles, including the jaw, become rigid and locked.

Many people associate stepping on a rusty nail with getting a tetanus shot, because the tetanus bacteria typically enter the body through wounds, including lacerations, punctures, scratches, animal bites, and cuts, especially those made by dirty or rusty objects. Because tetanus bacteria cannot live in the presence of oxygen, they thrive in deep wounds. Once in the body, the bacteria produce a poison that blocks the nerve signals allowing the muscles to relax. The result is extremely strong and painful muscle spasms that have the ability to break bones. Those who die of tetanus usually suffocate when the chest muscles become rigid.

Symptoms and Treatment

The first symptoms of tetanus are usually headache, chills, muscular stiffness of the jaw and neck, irritability, and fever. These occur one to three weeks after infection. They are followed by spasms and rigidity of the muscles: The legs and feet become extended, the arms stiffen, the hands clench, and the jaw is unable to open. As the stomach and chest muscles are affected, convulsions may occur and breathing becomes difficult.

Treatment of tetanus includes immediate injection with a tetanus antitoxin. Depending on how soon the shot is taken, people who have tetanus may also need antispasmodic drugs and tranquilizers. Complications of tetanus include pneumonia and bone fractures, which are caused by the tremendous pressure exerted on the bones from the rigid muscles.

Who Is at Risk for Tetanus?

Nearly all cases of tetanus in the United States occur in people who are fifty years and older and who have never been vaccinated or who have not had a tetanus booster shot within ten years of their injury. A tetanus shot should be given at the time of injury. If the wound is clean or minor, a booster may not be necessary if the individual had one within the past ten years. If the wound is dirty or contaminated, a booster shot should be given if more than five years have passed since the last shot.

Approximately fifty to one hundred cases of tetanus occur in the United States every year, and about 30 percent of them are fatal. The highest number of cases of tetanus ever reported in the United States was 601 in 1948. In 1992, there were forty-five cases and nine deaths. In 1999, forty cases were reported in the United States. Elsewhere, most cases of tetanus occur in underdeveloped countries that have poor sanitary conditions.

PERTUSSIS (WHOOPING COUGH)

Whooping cough, also known as the hundred-day cough, is a highly contagious disease that is caused by bacteria (*Bordetella pertussis*) found in the nose, throat, and mouth of infected individuals. Like diphtheria, it is spread through coughing, speaking, and sneezing. Most people who get whooping cough and recover acquire permanent immunity, although some people do get a milder case in the future.

The disease gets its name from the characteristic *whoop* sound children make as they struggle to breathe through blocked airways. The airways are blocked by a sticky mucus that is produced by the poisons released by the pertussis bacteria. The younger children are when they get whooping cough, the smaller are their air passages and therefore the more life threatening the disease can be.

Symptoms and Treatment

Within six to twenty days after exposure to whooping cough, symptoms begin to appear, starting with a short, dry, persistent cough. Because there is usually no fever, runny nose, or sore throat along with the cough, parents often think it is an allergic reaction. After ten to twelve days, mucus develops. The child usually has a low fever, coughs more at night, and may refuse to drink or eat.

The disease is most severe during the third and fourth week of infection, when severe coughing can cause the child to gag, vomit, and even stop breathing. Treatment includes the antibiotic erythromycin, which may help eliminate the infection and reduce the possibility of the disease spreading to others. However, neither over-the-counter cough and cold medications nor antibiotics appear to provide much relief, especially after the severe coughing has begun.

Infants and small children often need to be hospitalized during the worst few weeks of the disease in order to have the mucus suctioned out of their throats and to receive respiratory assistance. Children need to be watched closely for secondary infections that often accompany whooping cough, including pneumonia, ear infections, and bronchitis.

The entire course of whooping cough, including any secondary complications, usually lasts two to four months. Older children and adults also can get the disease because, even if they have been vaccinated, vaccine-acquired immunity wears off in later years. When older individuals do get whooping cough, it is often misdiagnosed as cold, flu, or bronchitis, especially since they do not have the *whoop* as a signal. Whooping cough in older children and adults is usually milder than it is in younger people, but it may be accompanied by bruised ribs, nosebleeds, and hemorrhaging in the eyes from the coughing.

Who Is at Risk for Whooping Cough?

Infants and young children up to one year of age are at the highest risk from the disease because they have the narrowest air passages and it is easy for mucus to block them. From 1990 to 1996, nearly 75 percent of infants younger than six months old who had the disease needed to be hospitalized, compared with less than 50 percent of those six months to one year of age and less than 20 percent of those one to four years of age.

Whooping cough is a cyclical disease with natural increases in countries around the world every three to four years. Although most cases of whooping cough are still reported in infants and children younger than ten years old, there is an increasing number of older children and adults getting the disease. This may be because it is recognized and diagnosed more often now than it was in the past, but there are also indications that the *B. pertussis* organism may be becoming vaccine-resistant. From 1985 to 1987, only 25 percent of all reported cases were in people older than ten years of age. This percentage leaped to 42 percent between 1995 and 1998. From 2000 to 2004, 2,488 cases were reported annually among infants younger than twelve months. There were 100 pertussis-related deaths.

THE DTP/DTaP VACCINE

The DTaP vaccine that is widely used today in the United States did not start out as a trio, or as DTaP. This vaccine's story begins with the first of the three vaccines to be developed— the pertussis vaccine, in 1906. The first pertussis vaccine was made using the whole-cell bacterium *Bordetella pertussis*. Then, as now, the vaccine was grown in a broth, and heat and chemicals were added to make the bacteria inactive. The bacteria are then placed in a solution that contains chemicals. Aluminum is added to help promote the production of antibodies.

The diphtheria vaccine was developed in the 1920s, and tetanus followed in 1933. Both vaccines are made similarly, but formaldehyde is used to detoxify the diphtheria and tetanus toxoids. This combination is then diluted with a solution that contains other preserving chemicals, and aluminum is added.

A Trio Is Born: DTP

In 1946, DTP—the first combination vaccine—was introduced to the US market. The DTP vaccine is an inactivated bacterial vaccine composed of the DT (diphtheria/tetanus) vaccine combined with whole-cell *B. pertussis* bacteria. For fifty years, DTP was the recommended vaccine for infants in the United States to prevent diphtheria, tetanus, and pertussis. But many years before the change to the new, safer DTaP vaccine was made in 1996, there were hints of problems with the vaccine— specifically with the pertussis portion, because that part of the vaccine included whole-cell bacteria, which were known to cause reactions. Serious adverse effects, including convulsions, shock, high fever, brain swelling, cardiac and respiratory distress, and brain damage, were being reported by mothers in countries where the vaccine was being used, including the United States, Europe, and Japan.

In response to several infant deaths after DTP in the 1970s, Japan, with the National Institutes of Health, took technology developed by Eli Lilly and refined it, creating a purified, less reactive acellular pertussis vaccine. Japan made the safer DTaP vaccine available to Japanese children in 1981, but the United States kept using the older, more dangerous form. This angered the mothers whose children were harmed by the whole-cell per-tussis vaccine in the DTP shot, so they took action.

The Fight for "New and Improved" DTaP

By the mid-1980s, approximately three hundred lawsuits had been filed against the manufacturers of the DTP vaccine. Among the hundreds of mothers whose children had experi-enced shock, convulsions, high fever, continuous crying, col-lapse, or brain damage after receiving one or more DTP shots was one whose son was left with attention deficit disorder and multiple learning disabilities after he had a severe reaction to his fourth DTP shot in 1980. That mother, Barbara Loe Fisher, joined with Kathi Williams and other parents whose children had experienced serious reactions to DTP and founded Dissatisfied Parents Together, which later became the National Vaccine Information Center. This national, nonprofit consumer advocacy organization was a driving force behind the introduction of the DTaP vaccine to the US market and the CDC's recommendation in 1996 that it be used instead of the DTP form.

The DTaP vaccine is made by removing many of the poisons (toxins) found in the whole-cell *B. pertussis* bacteria that are used in the DTP vaccine. What remains are just a few components of the bacteria rather than the whole organism. These components are detoxified using formaldehyde, and then aluminum is added. This acellular (rather than whole-cell) version of the pertussis vaccine is then combined with the DT vaccine to create DTaP.

Removing these toxins from pertussis also significantly reduces (but does not eliminate) the number and potency of the adverse effects associated with the vaccine. Unfortunately, DTaP was not made available to babies under eighteen months old in the United States until 1996.

How Effective Is DTP/DTaP Vaccine?

When DTP vaccine is given as recommended, the CDC claims that it protects more than 95 percent of the children against tetanus, more than 85 percent against diphtheria, and 70 to 90 percent against pertussis.

Researchers have also compared the efficacy of DTP and DTaP vaccines concerning the pertussis portions. They found the DTaP vaccine more effective in preventing moderate to severe pertussis, and that the DTaP form caused fewer adverse effects.

However, the effectiveness of the DTP/DTaP vaccines in

preventing pertussis overall has come into question. During the twenty years before the pertussis vaccine became available in the United States, 115,000 to nearly 270,000 cases of the disease were reported each year, with up to 10,000 deaths annually. From a high of 265,269 cases of whooping cough reported in the United States in 1934, the figure dropped to an all-time low of 1,010 cases in 1970. Between 1980 and 1998, the number of reported cases increased steadily. In 1993, for example, 6,586 cases were reported, more than in any year since 1976, and 6,279 cases were reported in 1998. In 2004, however, only 2,488 cases were reported in the United States. Some experts dispute these figures, however, saying that only 10 to 20 percent of all cases are being reported. Regardless of the accuracy of the total number of cases, the largest increase appears to be in people five years of age and older, but infants and young children still have the highest risk for the disease.

The experts are uncertain why pertussis cases increased even as the number of children being vaccinated with DTaP was greater than it had ever been. One reason may be that the vaccine's efficacy decreased; another is that immunity among children who have been vaccinated was declining over time, which may indicate the need for a booster shot. Other suggestions include an increased awareness of the disease by doctors, who then report it more often, or that states are monitoring the disease more closely. In any case, the recent numbers are decreasing.

There is some evidence that the *B. pertussis* bacteria are becoming resistant to the vaccine. Cases of whooping cough have broken out among vaccinated populations in Norway, Denmark, and the Netherlands, and scientists are finding more and more mutated strains of the bacteria.

FEDERAL/STATE GUIDELINES FOR DOSING OF DTP/DTaP

- Two months
- Four months
- Six months
- Twelve to eighteen months*
- Four to six years

*The fourth dose can be given as early as twelve months of age if at least six months have passed since the third dose and the child may not return at age fifteen to eighteen months.

Who Should Not Get the Vaccine?

According to the CDC, children who meet any of the following criteria should either not get the DTP or DTaP vaccine or wait. These are children who:

- Have had encephalopathy (brain inflammation/disease) within seven days of a previous dose of DTP or DTaP vaccine.
- Have a brain condition such as a seizure disorder that is not improving.
- Have experienced shock after DTP or DTaP.
- Have a moderate or severe illness and should wait until they have recovered.
- Are getting immunosuppressive therapy for cancer or other treatments. These children should wait until they are off such therapy for one month before getting the vaccine.
- Are younger than six weeks or older than seven years of age. Only the DT vaccine should be given (without the pertussis portion) after age seven. The DT vaccine can also be given

to some younger children who have had an adverse reaction to the pertussis portion of the DTP or DTaP vaccine.

The following conditions are considered "precautions" by the CDC:

- Fever of 105 degrees or greater within forty-eight hours of a previous DTP or DTaP shot.
- Collapse or shock within forty-eight hours of a DTP or DTaP shot.
- Seizures with or without fever within seventy-two hours of a DTP or DTaP shot.
- Persistent inconsolable crying lasting three or more days within forty-eight hours of a DTP or DTaP shot.

ADVERSE REACTIONS

The CDC lists the following reactions as being associated with the DTaP vaccine. According to the Vaccine Adverse Events Reporting System (VAERS), adverse events associated with the older DTP vaccine are 30 percent greater overall than those listed below. Thus introduction of the DTaP vaccine has resulted in a significant reduction in adverse reactions. If mild reactions occur, they usually begin within three days of receiving the vaccine and disappear within a few days.

Common mild reactions include:

- Pain or soreness at the injection site: 46 out of 1,000 children.
- Low fever: 58 out of 1,000 children.
- Fussiness: 300 out of 1,000 children.
- Swelling: 80 out of 1,000 children.

Moderate to serious reactions, which are more uncommon, include the following:

- High-pitched screaming or continuous crying for three or more hours: 1 out of 2,000 children (1 per 100 doses).
- High fever (greater than 105 degrees): 1 out of 3,000 children (1 per 330 doses).
- Seizures (jerking or staring): 6 out of every 10,000 doses (1 per 1,750 doses).
- Child is pale, limp, less alert: 6 out of every 10,000 doses (1 per 1,750 doses).

Cases of severe adverse effects, says the CDC, are very rare and include severe allergic reactions (difficulty breathing, shock) and severe brain reaction (brain inflammation, coma, reduced consciousness, or a long seizure). The CDC also claims that although fever accompanied by seizures after DTP/DTaP shots is frightening to parents, there is no evidence that this reaction causes any permanent damage. The CDC does, however, acknowledge a link between DTP and the serious brain disease encephalopathy. The National Childhood Encephalopathy Study published in Britain in 1981, and reconfirmed in 1991, found that 1 in 110,000 DTP shots is followed by a brain inflammation and 1 in 310,000 DTP shots is followed by permanent brain damage.

Precautions from the Manufacturers

The product inserts that vaccine manufacturers include with their products contain more precautions than those listed by the CDC. For that reason, and because the manufacturers often update these inserts, you are encouraged to ask your doctor for a copy of the manufacturer's product information during the visit *before* the vaccination occurs. Barbara Loe Fisher's National Vaccine Information Center reports:

• At least one DTaP vaccine manufacturer admitted on its product insert statement that DTaP "has not been evaluated for carcinogenic [cancer-causing], mutagenic [causing mutations] potentials or impairment of fertility."
• "Hypersensitivity to any component of the vaccine, including thimerosal, a mercury derivative, is a contraindication."
• Referring to DTaP: "Influenza virus vaccine should not be given within three days of the administration of [the vaccine]."

SERIOUS REACTIONS: WHAT TO LOOK FOR, WHAT TO DO

Moderate or severe health problems following the DTP/DTaP vaccine should be reported to and checked by a doctor immediately. All adverse events that occur within thirty days of any vaccination should also be reported to the Vaccine Adverse Events Reporting System (VAERS), which is explained in chapter 22. DTP/DTaP reaction signs to look for include:

• Anaphylaxis/shock (difficulty breathing, wheezing, fast heartbeat, dizziness, hives, weakness)
• Seizure (twitching, jerking, staring, stiffness)
• Difficulty breathing
• Paleness/limpness
• Coma or lowered consciousness

Side Effects of DT, Td, Tdap, and Tetanus Vaccines

Children older than ten years and adults who get the Tdap booster shots and tetanus toxoid shots may also experience side effects from the injections. They include pain and swelling at the injection site, irritability, vomiting, sleepiness, loss of appetite, persistent crying, fever, collapse, rash, joint pain, cold skin, and paleness.

The absence of the pertussis portion of the vaccine does not exclude the DT, Td, or tetanus vaccines from the possibility of causing serious adverse effects. In 1994, the Institute of Medicine reported that there is compelling proof that DT vaccine can cause brachial neuritis, a neuropathy, and Guillain-Barré syndrome, a condition characterized by progressive deterioration of the muscles, nerve inflammation, shock, and death. Unfortunately, there are no studies to determine whether these vaccines may be associated with multiple sclerosis and other demyelinating diseases, arthritis, and seizure disorders.

THE TROUBLE WITH DTP

In her 1985 book *A Shot in the Dark,* Barbara Loe Fisher reveals the story of the DTP vaccine, and describes hundreds of cases of children who suffered symptoms after receiving the vaccine, and why the safer DTaP vaccine was withheld from the US market until 1996. Now, of course, DTaP is in wide use. Parents should always ask the health care provider giving the vaccine whether their child is getting the DTaP form of the vaccine.

When parents across America (and around the world) began clamoring for more information about and investigation into adverse reactions to DTP, they found that few studies had ever been done to determine if the vaccine was linked to serious health problems. But the parents were seeing certain problems in their children: seizures, anemia, attention deficit disorder, aseptic meningitis, Guillain-Barré syndrome, juvenile diabetes, learning disabilities, and thrombocytopenia (low number of blood platelets, which leads to abnormal bleeding). Because of these parents' efforts, medical experts began to take a closer look at DTP. Here are some of the things they found.

- In 1991, experts at the Institute of Medicine determined that there was compelling evidence that DTP vaccine caused acute inflammation of the brain (encephalopathy, encephalitis, encephalomyelitis), shock, collapse, and prolonged, continuous crying.
- A 1991 study of sudden infant death syndrome (SIDS) monitored episodes of shallow and stopped breathing in infants both before and after they received DTP. The breathing patterns were printed out by computer and showed that the vaccinations caused a significant increase in episodes where breathing either stopped completely or nearly did so. These episodes continued for several months. The author of the study, Dr. Viera Scheibner, stated that "vaccination is the single most prevalent and most preventable cause of infant deaths" (see chapter 5).
- A 1992 study found that infants die at a rate eight times greater than normal within three days of receiving a DTP shot.
- A 1994 study found that children with asthma were five times more likely than not to have received the pertussis vaccine.

- In 1994, the Institute of Medicine reported that "some children who receive DTP and who experience a serious acute neurologic illness within 7 days thereafter would be expected to go on to experience chronic nervous system dysfunction or die."
- In August 1999, Marcel Kinsbourne, M.D., of Tufts University, told members of the Committee on Government Reform that "it is well known that some lots of pertussis vaccine are associated with a disproportionately high number of notifications of adverse events." In fact, more than half the adverse events reported to the Vaccine Adverse Events Reporting System (VAERS) concern DTP.

BOTTOM LINE

Combination vaccines always send up a red flag for me, and DTaP is no exception. Although the newer DTaP vaccine is safer than the older DTP form, the pertussis portion of both vaccines seems to still be causing serious adverse reactions in some children. But even the diphtheria and tetanus portions of the vaccine are problematic, as the Institute of Medicine concluded in 1994 (see above).

So where does that leave you as a parent who is concerned about giving the vaccine to your child? Carefully go over the list of "Who Should Not Get the Vaccine?" in this chapter before you allow your child to get the shot. If your child does not fit into any of those categories and you still wish to proceed, I suggest that your child not get the shot along with any other vaccine that day. That way, if there are any complications, you will know which vaccine caused the problem. Also, follow the suggestions listed at the end of chapter 21. Together these precautions can help maximize chances your child will fare well with the DTaP vaccine.

NOTES

Auwaeter, P. G., et al. "Changes Within T Cell Receptor V-beta Subsets in Infants Following Measles Vaccination." *Clinical Immunology and Immunopathology* 79, no. 2 (May 1996): 163–70.

Centers for Disease Control and Prevention. Vaccine Information Statements. May 4, 2000.

CureResearch.com Web site: www.cureresearch.com.

Fine, J. M., and L. C. Chen. "Confounding in Studies of Adverse Reactions to Vaccines." *American Journal of Epidemiology* 136 (1992): 121–35.

Fisher, Barbara Loe. *The Consumer's Guide to Childhood Vaccines.* Vienna, VA: National Vaccine Information Center, 1997, 10, 37, 36, 56.

Humiston, Sharon G., and Cynthia Good. *Vaccinating Your Child: Questions and Answers for the Concerned Parent.* Atlanta: Peachtree Publishers, 2000, 79, 81, 85.

de Melker, H. E., et al. "Reemergence of Pertussis in the Highly Vaccinated Population of the Netherlands: Observations on Surveillance Data." *Emergent Infectious Diseases* 6, no. 4 (July–August 2000): 348–57.

Odent, Michael, et al. "Pertussis Vaccination and Asthma: Is There a Link?" *Journal of the American Medical Association* 272, no. 8 (August 1994): 592–93.

Pertussis.com Web site: www.pertussis.com.

Scheibner, Viera, and Leif Karlsson. "Association Between Non-Specific Stress Syndrome, DPT Injections, and Cot Death." Second Immunization Conference, Canberra, Australia, May 27–29, 1991.

Sheldon, T. "Dutch Whooping Cough Epidemic Puzzles Scientists." *British Medical Journal* 316 (January 10, 1998): 92.

Van Boven, M., and H. E. de Melker. "Waning Immunity and Sub-Clinical Infection in an Epidemic Model: Implications for Pertussis in the Netherlands." *Mathematical Biosciences* 164, no. 2 (April 2000): 161–82.

www.cdc.gov/travel/yellowbook/2008/ch4/hep-b.aspx.

Chapter 8

❁

Hib: *Haemophilus Influenzae* Type B Vaccine

THE HIB (*HAEMOPHILUS INFLUENZAE* TYPE B) VACCINE WAS developed to help eliminate a disease that at one time affected about twenty thousand children per year in the United States and was responsible for about five hundred deaths annually. If Hib disease does not sound familiar to you, perhaps bacterial meningitis does. Bacterial meningitis is the most common complication of this bacterial disease. It is the reason the Hib vaccine is sometimes called the meningitis vaccine, even though it is effective against only one of the many types of meningitis.

You may think from the name *influenzae* that Hib disease has something to do with the flu, but it doesn't. The doctor who named the disease back in 1892, Dr. Pfeiffer, mistakenly thought the bacteria was associated with the influenza epidemic that was occurring at the time. Although scientists cleared up the mistake in the 1930s, they decided to keep the name.

In this chapter you will learn about Hib disease and the

"meningitis vaccine," and why the CDC believes children in the United States should receive this vaccine.

HIB DISEASE

Hib disease is a contagious condition caused by the bacterium *Haemophilus influenzae* type B. It is spread through contact with mucus or droplets from the nose or throat, as when people cough, kiss, sneeze, or share personal items like drinking cups and toothbrushes. The infection is carried by nose and throat excretions into the bloodstream and then settles into various parts of the body, often the spinal fluid and the brain.

Who Gets Hib Disease?

During the early part of the twentieth century, it was rare to see Hib disease in newborns and adults. Then between 1946 and 1986, there was a fourfold increase in the disease among these two groups. Although scientists are uncertain why this increase occurred, one theory is that the excessive use of antibiotics forced the bacteria to mutate and become more resistant.

Since the introduction of Hib vaccine in 1985, the disease is most commonly seen in children between the ages of two months and three years, with the peak time being at six to seven months of age. It only infrequently occurs in people older than five years of age. The number of cases is down dramatically, however: In 1998, only 228 cases of Hib disease were reported in children in the United States, a 99 percent decrease from the approximately 20,000 of just a few decades ago, due in part to the vaccine.

Even though cases of Hib disease in people older than five years of age are rare, they do occur. Three out of 1,000 people who come into close contact with a child who has Hib disease will get the disease. Given that there are so few cases of Hib in the United States, the risk is extremely slight. People who are at increased risk of getting Hib disease include:

- Blacks, Hispanics, and Native Americans, who get the disease more than do whites.
- People with chronic diseases, such as cancer and sickle-cell anemia.
- Children who are in close contact with other children, especially in day care settings, where there are children in the high-risk years.
- Males, who get the disease more often than do females.

Symptoms

Hib disease can cause several different complications (discussed below), depending on the area of the body the bacteria invade. The most common symptoms that signal infection with *H. influenzae* include high fever, headache, vomiting, and a stiff back or neck. Symptoms usually appear in less than ten days, and most often within two to four days after someone has been exposed to the disease. Infants who have Hib disease cannot tell you they have a headache or a stiff neck; therefore caregivers should be on the lookout for Hib disease if they see symptoms that include irritability, inactivity, poor feeding, and vomiting.

Hib meningitis is diagnosed by examining a sample of the spinal fluid. People who have Hib disease can continue to spread it to others as long as the bacteria are in their throat and nose, even if their symptoms have disappeared. They are no longer contagious after taking antibiotics for one to two days.

Unlike some other contagious diseases, such as measles and

chicken pox, in which having the disease allows people to develop a natural immunity to it (see "Two Types of Immunity" in chapter 1), not all children who have had Hib disease are so protected. Some children, especially those who have a compromised (weak) immune system, can get a repeat Hib infection.

Complications of Hib Disease

Hib disease is the most common cause of bacterial meningitis in the United States, accounting for 50 to 65 percent of all Hib cases. Other complications include epiglottitis, septic arthritis, cellulitis, pneumonia, osteomyelitis, and bacteremia.

- **Bacterial meningitis**: Bacterial meningitis is an infection of the brain and spinal cord coverings that most often affects children aged six months to four years. It can be caused by several different types of bacteria: type B (*H. influenzae*), meningococcal (*Neisseria meningitidis*), and pneumococcal (*Pneumococcus* spp.). The Hib vaccine is designed to prevent type B only.

  Symptoms of bacterial meningitis include high fever, headache, a stiff neck, and loss of appetite. Five to 10 percent of infected individuals die. Between 15 and 20 percent of the children who recover from the disease develop epilepsy, mental retardation, heart damage, deafness, or blindness. Serious Hib disease is only found in 1.3 / 100,000 children in the United States presently due to the use of the vaccine.

  Not everyone who has *H. influenzae* bacteria gets meningitis. In fact, up to 90 percent of healthy people harbor the bacteria in their respiratory tract, where it lies dormant for their entire lives.

- **Epiglottitis:** This infection affects the epiglottis, a leaf-shaped flap in the throat where the food pipe (esophagus) and windpipe (trachea) meet. The infection can cause the epiglottis to swell to the point that it causes asphyxiation. Children with epiglottitis gasp when they inhale, which causes them to lean forward in an attempt to breathe better. Epiglottitis affects about 15 percent of children with Hib disease.

- **Septic arthritis:** Fever accompanied by redness, pain, and swelling of a joint are the signs of septic arthritis, an infection that can destroy the affected joint. It occurs in about 12 percent of children who have Hib disease.
- **Cellulitis:** This skin infection causes fever, redness, swelling, and pain, usually of the face, neck, or head. About 10 pecent of children with Hib disease develop this complication. Cellulitis can be life threatening if the infection spreads to the brain.
- **Pneumonia:** About 15 percent of children with Hib disease develop this infection of the lungs. Signs and symptoms include fever, cough, and difficulty breathing.
- **Osteomyelitis:** This infection of the bone can destroy the bone if the infection penetrates deeply, causing the bone to stop growing. Signs and symptoms include fever, swelling, redness, and pain in the affected limb. It occurs in only about 3 to 4 percent of Hib disease cases.
- **Bacteremia:** About 2 to 3 percent of children with Hib disease develop this blood infection. This complication can be life threatening if it spreads to the brain.

THE HIB VACCINE

The *Haemophilus influenzae* type B bacteria was first isolated from victims of an influenza epidemic in 1892, which is when it was incorrectly identified as an "influenza." It wasn't until nearly one hundred years later that a vaccine for the bacterial infection was developed.

Recognition of the need for a Hib vaccine became apparent in 1933, when researchers realized that most cases of Hib meningitis were occurring in children younger than five years of age. Scientists at the time were unable to create an adequate vaccine, however, and so when antibiotics became widely available in the 1950s and 1960s and greatly reduced the death rate from meningitis, they thought they were getting a handle on the disease.

Yet follow-up studies showed that children who recovered from Hib meningitis often had severe problems, including mental retardation and epilepsy. The need for a vaccine became more urgent. Back in the laboratory, investigators created several vaccines. The first Hib vaccine was on the market only from 1983 to 1985 because researchers discovered that it was not effective in children younger than eighteen months, its performance in older children was uncertain, and in some cases it was causing Hib meningitis. So they returned to the laboratory.

In 1987, researchers developed a new form of the vaccine, conjugate Hib. This vaccine was effective in infants and children and was licensed in 1990. In January 1991, the CDC recommended that it be part of the childhood routine immunization schedule. Their rationale was that among unvaccinated children aged two months to three years, antibody levels against *H. influenzae* are minimal. Therefore children younger than three years are the most vulnerable and thus need to be immunized.

How Effective Is the Vaccine?

The vaccine is reportedly at least 95 percent effective in children who receive all the shots in the series. Depending on which brand of vaccine your child receives, the series may include three or four shots.

Since introduction of the Hib conjugate vaccine, incidence of the disease among children aged four years and younger has declined 98 percent. About three hundred cases of the disease occur each year in the United States, most of them in unimmunized children and most caused by non-type-B *H. influenzae.*

VACCINATION RECOMMENDATION

According to Ronald Kennedy, Ph.D., professor of microbiology at the University of Oklahoma Health Sciences Center, the combination vaccine of Hib, hepatitis B, and DTP may render the hepatitis B inactive. I would suggest that in light of this, you avoid this vaccine schedule and get the vaccines separately on different days. Also note that the vaccine should be injected into the muscles of the upper arm or thigh.

Adverse Reactions

The CDC reports that up to 25 percent of children who get the Hib vaccine experience minor pain, redness, or swelling at the injection site. About 5 percent of children develop a fever or irritability within a few hours of receiving the vaccination. These minor problems usually resolve within two to three days.

Moderate to severe reactions are rare and include high fever, behavioral changes, and serious allergic reactions that include hives, difficulty breathing, hoarseness, fast heart rate, dizziness, or wheezing within a few minutes to a few hours after receiving the vaccine.

More serious side effects of the Hib vaccine have been reported by parents, including thrombocytopenia (abnormal decrease in the number of blood platelets), Guillain-Barré syndrome, insulin-dependent diabetes, and an increase in Hib disease. According to an August 2000 study, however, researchers say there is no link between Hib vaccine and diabetes (see chapter 5).

FEDERAL/STATE GUIDELINES FOR HIB VACCINE DOSING

According to the CDC:

- Children should get the Hib vaccine at two months, four months, six months, and twelve to fifteen months of age.
- If you miss a dose or do not follow the schedule, get the next dose as soon as possible. You do not need to start the series again.
- Hib vaccine may be given at the same time as other vaccines. Many experts, including myself, do not recommend giving more than one vaccine at a time (except Hib and IPV), see chapter 21. Simultaneous injections (also known as multiple dosing) not only increase the chance of adverse reactions, but if problems do occur, it will be virtually impossible to know which vaccine or ingredient caused them.

Who Should Not Get the Vaccine?

The CDC recommends that people who fall into any of the following categories should not get the vaccine, or should delay it:

- Anyone older than five years of age usually does not need the Hib vaccine. Exceptions include individuals who have sickle-cell disease or HIV/AIDS; those who have had their spleen removed or a bone marrow transplant; and those who have received or are receiving drug treatment for cancer. Anyone in these categories should discuss the possible need for Hib vaccine with their doctor.
- Anyone who has ever had a life-threatening reaction to a previous Hib dose.
- Anyone who is moderately or severely ill at the time the shot is scheduled.
- Infants younger than six weeks of age.

SERIOUS REACTIONS: WHAT TO LOOK FOR, WHAT TO DO

According to the CDC, moderate or severe reactions to Hib vaccine should be reported to and checked by a doctor immediately. If any of these reactions were to occur they would happen within a few minutes to a few hours after receiving the shot. All adverse reactions should also be reported to the Vaccine Adverse Events Reporting System (VAERS), explained in chapter 22. Signs to look for include:

- High fever
- Behavior changes
- Difficulty breathing
- Hoarseness or wheezing
- Weakness
- Fast heartbeat
- Dizziness
- Hives
- Paleness

BOTTOM LINE

The Hib vaccine appears to cause fewer problems than other mandated childhood vaccines, yet it is not without its risks. Over a million doses of Hib vaccine were recalled in 2007 after sterility testing at a Merck facility revealed contamination with a bacterium, *Bacillus cereus*. Dr. Julie Gerberding, former head of the CDC, said, "This is not a health threat in the short run, but it is an inconvenience." I would consider this a health threat if these contaminated vaccines had been injected into children.

As with all vaccines, I urge you to carefully read the information about who should not get the vaccine and to only allow your child to get the vaccine if he or she is well on the day the shot is scheduled, unless your doctor advises otherwise. In addition, follow the "Actions Parents Can Take" at the end of chapter 21 to help ensure your child will be protected against any possible adverse reactions to the vaccine.

NOTES

Centers for Disease Control and Prevention. Vaccine Information Statements. May 4, 2000.

Fisher, Barbara Loe. *The Consumer's Guide to Childhood Vaccines.* Vienna, VA: National Vaccine Information Center, 1997, 20, 30, 42ff.

Humiston, Sharon G., and Cynthia Good. *Vaccinating Your Child: Questions and Answers for the Concerned Parent.* Atlanta: Peachtree Publishers, 2000, 101–7.

National Institute of Allergy and Infectious Diseases Web site: www .niaid.nih.gov/publications/economic/vaccine.htm.

"No Link Between Hib or Hepatitis B and Diabetes or Crohn's Disease," at www.usatoday.com/life/health/child/lhchi204.htm.

www.en.wikipedia.org/wiki/Haemophilus_influenza.

Chapter 9

❖

Polio

IF YOU ARE A LATE BABY BOOMER OR YOUNGER, CHANCES ARE you don't have any peers who have had polio. If you are of a more mature age (or a history buff), you may remember that President Franklin Delano Roosevelt governed the country from his wheelchair, a permanent reminder to him and the nation that he was a victim of this crippling disease.

Roosevelt contracted the disease long before the introduction of the first polio vaccine in 1955. Now, thankfully, polio cases are rare. In 1985, the World Health Organization (WHO) declared that one of its goals was global elimination of polio by the year 2000. Although it fell a bit short of its goal globally (several thousand cases were reported in 1999 in Africa, Southeast Asia, and the eastern Mediterranean), no cases of natural polio have been reported in the entire Western Hemisphere since 1991.

Yet although the risk of acquiring natural ("wild") polio (catching it from another person) is virtually nil in the United States, the chances of getting it through a vaccine are not. During

1980 to 1985, fifty-five cases of paralytic polio were reported; four cases were brought into the country by travelers who had it naturally, and fifty-one cases were caused by the live vaccine.

As of January 1, 2000, the oral form of the vaccine, which has been identified as causing the disease, is no longer recommended for use in the United States, except in limited circumstances. Instead, the killed injectable polio vaccine (IPV), which has been available longer than the oral form, is recommended.

Even as the cases of polio fade from the world, the controversies surrounding the polio vaccines do not. That's why in this chapter we discuss not only the disease polio and the recommended use of the two vaccines, but also the debates about the use of monkey kidney cultures to make the vaccine and the possible links between polio vaccine and HIV/AIDS or cancer.

POLIO

Polio, also known as poliomyelitis, is believed to have a very long history. Ancient Egyptian drawings show people with shriveled limbs, a characteristic of this viral disease, which destroys the nerve cells in the spinal cord and brain stem, causing paralysis and atrophy of the arms and legs. If the virus attacks the part of the spinal cord that controls breathing, it can cause death.

The only way to catch the wild polio virus is from an infected person. The virus is found in the stools, and it enters the body through the mouth. This is one reason why infants and young children are the ones most commonly affected, as they tend to explore their world with their mouths and hands. Fecal contamination is common in environments where infants and children are present, such as in day care centers. Noncontaminated adults can pass along the virus if they don't wash their hands after changing the diaper of an infected child.

When the virus enters the body, it reproduces in the throat and intestines and attacks the lymph nodes and blood. Once the virus is in the blood, it sometimes travels to the central nervous system and destroys the brain stem and spinal nerves, leading to permanent paralysis.

Who Gets Polio?

Polio is still found in Southeast Asia (58 percent of cases), Africa (21 percent), and the eastern Mediterranean (21 percent). In countries where polio still occurs, it affects more children than adults, but adults are more likely to become paralyzed by the disease. More adults also die of the disease: 15 to 30 percent of affected adults compared with 2 to 5 percent of children.

Since 1979, there have been no cases of natural (wild) polio in the United States other than four cases that were brought into the country by travelers.

Symptoms

About 95 percent of the people who become infected with the polio virus do not have major symptoms and recover without permanent damage, but they are carriers and can pass it along through their stools. Before nerve damage occurs in those who are seriously affected by the virus, sore throat, nausea, or fever typically occur. Then as the nerves become affected, people become weak and experience abnormal sensations, usually in the arms or legs. As the nerve damage progresses, the muscles in the affected areas shrink and become paralyzed. If the diaphragm is involved, breathing is affected.

When Is Polio Not Polio?

The introduction of the polio vaccines in 1955 and 1961 is generally credited with causing a dramatic decline in the number of polio cases in the United States. In fact, compared with the more than twenty thousand people a year who were developing paralytic polio by the early 1950s, the number was only sixty-one by 1965.

But was this dramatic drop in the number of polio cases all due to the vaccines? Or was it the result of manipulation of the statistics and redefinition of nonparalytic poliomyelitis and viral meningitis, a disease with symptoms very similar to those of polio?

After the Salk polio vaccine was introduced in the United States, two significant changes were made in how the disease was classified. First, the term *paralytic poliomyelitis* was redefined to include those who had paralysis for at least sixty days rather than the mere twenty-four hours required previously. This greatly reduced the number of cases classified as polio and added the cases that would formerly be placed in the polio category into the meningitis category.

Second, for reporting purposes, doctors were to make a distinction between aseptic meningitis and poliomyelitis rather than combine the diseases into one category. This change also resulted in a significant decline in the number of reported polio cases and a large increase in the number of meningitis cases.

Polio Vaccine: Why?

Because these changes occurred soon after the vaccine was introduced, the statistics for polio appear to support the claims that the vaccine was responsible for the decline in the number of cases. However, critics say that the decline would have occurred anyway, given the new definitions. To be fair, the vaccines have had a positive effect on the incidence of polio, but exactly how much is not known.

The bigger question today is, assuming a lesser role for immunization in bringing down polio rates, and the fact that natural polio has been gone from the United States for decades, why is the vaccine still required? The answer given by federal health officials is that the disease is still common in some parts of the world. Thus, notes the Vaccine Information Statement for the polio vaccine, "it would only take one case of polio from another country to bring the disease back if we were not protected by vaccine."

Some critics, however, say that federal officials and vaccine manufacturers are treating the polio vaccine as they did the smallpox vaccine. In that situation, the "smallpox vaccination remained the only source of smallpox-related deaths for three decades after the disease had disappeared" from the world. Does this sound familiar?

POLIO VACCINE

Although it appears that polio has been around for more than two thousand years, large outbreaks did not appear until the early 1800s, first in Europe and then throughout developing countries, such as the United States and Canada. The first large-scale epidemic in the United States occurred in 1916, when more than twenty-seven thousand people contracted the disease and about six thousand died. The majority of the victims were children.

The medical community became alarmed, and the search for the cause of polio, and a cure, was on. Speculations that polio was caused by an airborne germ, was carried by mosquitoes, or was brought to the United States by immigrants were all proved incorrect in 1908. Then in the late 1940s and early

1950s, John Enders, Thomas Weller, and their research team at Harvard University discovered that polioviruses (there are three different viruses) are transmitted through fecal matter—hands that touch infected fecal matter while changing diapers, and so on.

What scientists also discovered about polio was that it was more common among children who lived in sanitary conditions than those who lived in unsanitary ones because in the latter group, the children are more likely to get the virus at a young age as a carrier and develop immunity to it. The later in life people contract the poliovirus, the less likely the immune system is prepared to fight it.

POLIO VACCINE—A QUICK HISTORY

Circa 1908: Karl Landsteiner is the first to identify polio as a viral disease. He induces polio in monkeys.

1910: The first inactivated polio vaccine is developed by Paul Heinrich Romer, but it fails when Romer's subjects (monkeys) get polio.

Early 1930s: The two vaccines—one inactivated and one live—are developed, but by 1935 they prove to cause paralytic poliomyelitis and are withdrawn.

1930s: Scientists discover that polio is caused by various strains of poliovirus.

1949: Monkey kidney tissue becomes the preferred culture for growing polio vaccine.

1951: Scientists complete classification of polioviruses and identify three types. The cost of the project: $1,370,000 and the lives of thirty thousand monkeys.

1954: Jonas Salk develops an inactivated polio vaccine (IPV).

1954–1962: As many as thirty million Americans are possibly given IPV that has been contaminated with a monkey (simian) virus known as SV40, which has been linked with cancer; see "Polio Vaccine and Cancer" in this chapter. Not until 1961 are manufacturers required to test for SV40.

1955: In April, several months after 400,000 children receive the IPV made by Cutter Laboratories, 360 children become paralyzed from the vaccine. The polio virus was not fully killed before the vaccine was released.

1960: Albert Sabin develops a live oral polio vaccine (OPV).

2000: The CDC no longer recommends the oral polio vaccine except in limited circumstances.

The Birth of Two Polio Vaccines

By the early 1950s, more than twenty thousand cases of polio a year were reported in the United States. The need for a vaccine was critical, as Americans were haunted by the sight of rows and rows of children in iron lungs, the tomb-like machines that kept them alive by breathing for them because their diaphragms had been paralyzed by poliovirus.

Jonas Salk and his research team were the first to come to the rescue. In 1953, they announced an injectable polio vaccine (IPV) composed of poliovirus killed by formaldehyde, and in 1955 a mass immunization program began. The IPV was modified in 1987, and this newer version is used today. It is made using three types of poliovirus grown in cultures of African green monkey kidney cells. The viruses are made inactive with formaldehyde. The vaccine also contains phenoxyethanol as a preservative and three antibiotics—neomycin, streptomycin, and polymyxin B.

On Salk's heels was Dr. Albert Sabin, with his team, who developed an oral polio vaccine (OPV) that was licensed in 1961. It became much more widely used because it was painless (the vaccine was put into sugar cubes and ingested), less expensive than Salk's vaccine, and thought to be more effective because it not only vaccinated the recipient but also "passively vaccinated" those who came in close contact with a recently vaccinated person. It also could be given by nonmedical personnel, which made it easy to give in remote areas of the world.

Unlike Sabin's vaccine, Salk's vaccine contains live viruses. Once they enter a person's body, they reproduce rapidly, providing immunity more quickly than the injectable, inactivated vaccine. The oral form contains three types of weakened polio viruses grown in African green monkey kidney cell culture. The resulting cells are then grown in a solution of calf serum, amino acids, and antibiotics. After the cells have grown, the solution is removed and replaced with the virus. The vaccine also contains streptomycin, neomycin, and sorbitol.

How Effective Are the Polio Vaccines?

The oral polio vaccine provides immunity for 50 percent of people after one dose and 95 percent after three doses. Lifetime immunity is achieved after receiving the full series of four doses. However, the oral vaccine has also been shown to cause polio— about ten cases per year—and so after January 1, 2000, it was no longer recommended for use in the United States except in limited circumstances.

The injectable polio vaccine provides immunity for 90

percent of people after two doses and 99 percent after three. Lifetime immunity, however, is questionable. For that reason, France, which has used IPV almost exclusively for many years, gives booster shots to adults. The United States now recommends IPV for most people.

FEDERAL/STATE DOSING FOR POLIO VACCINE

According to the CDC, IPV should be given on the following schedule:

IPV

- Children: at two months, four months, six to eighteen months, and a booster dose at four to six years.
- Children who have already received one or more OPV doses can finish their series with IPV.
- Adults: The CDC recommends the vaccine for adults who meet the following criteria: those who plan to travel to polio-infected areas, those who handle lab specimens that may contain poliovirus, those who are in close contact with patients who may be passing the virus in their stool, and anyone who lives in a community where there is a polio outbreak. Their vaccination schedule should be: the first dose at any time, the second one to two months later, and the third six to twelve months after the second. The vaccine may be given either just under the skin or injected into the upper arm or thigh muscles.
- Adults who have had one or two doses of polio vaccine in the past (OPV or IPV) should get the remaining

one or two doses, regardless of how long it has been since they got the earlier dose(s).

- Adults who have had three or more doses of polio vaccine (OPV or IPV) in the past may need a booster. Ask your health care provider.

OPV

The limited circumstances under which OPV can be given include:

- Mass immunization to control an outbreak of polio.
- Children who have not yet received their first polio dose and who will be traveling within four weeks to a region of the world where polio is common. Only the first dose should be OPV.
- Anyone who has a life-threatening allergy to the antibiotics in the IPV vaccine—neomycin, streptomycin, or polymyxin B, or anyone who has had a life-threatening allergic reaction to IPV. *Note:* Despite this recommendation by the CDC, the oral polio vaccine does contain two of these antibiotics (neomycin and streptomycin) and so should not be recommended for individuals with life-threatening allergies, either.

Who Should Not Get the Vaccine?

The CDC recommends that anyone who meets the following criteria should either not get IPV or should wait:

- Anyone who has ever had a life-threatening allergic reaction to neomycin, streptomycin, or polymyxin B.

- Anyone who has had a severe allergic reaction to a previous polio vaccine dose.
- Anyone who is moderately or severely ill when the shot is scheduled should wait until they have recovered. *Note:* I personally recommend that people with minor illnesses, such as a cold, should also wait until they recover to be vaccinated because their immune system is compromised.

The CDC recommends that anyone who meets the following criteria should not get the OPV. Now that this vaccine is used in only very limited situations, these recommendations apply to a small number of people.

- Anyone who is taking long-term steroids or any other drug that affects the immune system.
- Anyone who has AIDS, HIV infection, or any other immune system disease.
- Anyone who has cancer or is getting chemotherapy.
- If anyone in the previous three groups changes an infant's diapers or has close contact with a child who is getting polio vaccine, that child should not get OPV.
- Anyone who has had a severe allergic reaction to a previous dose of OPV.
- Infants should not get OPV if anyone who will be in close contact with them has never had any polio vaccine.
- Anyone who is moderately or severely ill at the time the dose is scheduled should wait until he or she has recovered to receive the dose. *Note:* I recommend that people who have even a minor illness wait.

Adverse Reactions

The Vaccine Information Statement (VIS) given to those who are getting IPV states that most people have no adverse reactions to IPV and that there have never been any serious problems. Minor reactions include soreness or redness at the injection site for about 13 percent of people. Fever of 102 degrees or higher is reported in 38 percent of cases. There are, however, major concerns about the polio vaccines, as noted below under "Polio Vaccine and AIDS" and "Polio Vaccine and Cancer."

The VIS for the oral polio vaccine notes that it has caused several cases of polio every year it has been given (about 1 case for every 2.4 million doses of vaccine), which is the reason the vaccine is no longer recommended. Between 1980 and 1994, a total of 125 people developed vaccine-associated paralytic polio.

SERIOUS REACTIONS:
WHAT TO LOOK FOR, WHAT TO DO

According to the CDC, moderate or severe reactions to polio vaccines should be reported to and checked by a doctor immediately. Then she or he can determine the course of action. Signs to look for include:

- High fever
- Behavior changes
- Difficulty breathing
- Hoarseness or wheezing
- Weakness
- Fast heartbeat
- Dizziness

- Hives
- Paleness
- Swelling of the throat
- Paralysis (after OPV)

If any of these reactions except paralysis were to occur, they would happen within a few minutes to a few hours after receiving the shot. If paralysis were to occur after OPV, it could happen from about a week up to a month after the dose was given. Any reaction should be reported to the Vaccine Adverse Events Reporting System (VAERS). Ask your doctor, nurse, or health department to file the VAERS form for you, or you can call VAERS at 800-822-7967.

POLIO VACCINE AND AIDS

For years there have been reports circulating that the virus that causes AIDS (acquired immunodeficiency syndrome) was originally transferred from chimpanzees or monkeys to humans when the OPV was undergoing testing. Edward Hooper, author of *The River: A Journey to the Source of HIV and AIDS,* believes that the experimental OPV was produced using chimpanzee tissues that were infected with an HIV-related monkey virus. That contaminated vaccine was allegedly given to children who were living in what was then the Belgian Congo (now Burundi, the Congo, and Rwanda) beginning in 1957, when the first mass oral polio vaccine campaign was initiated. Within three years, 325,000 Africans were vaccinated in an area that is now considered to be the center of the AIDS epidemic.

The allegations of contamination have been denied by the physicians who conducted the trials, Drs. Stanley Plotkin and

Hilary Koprowski, who claim that they did not use chimpanzee tissue. They also state that the probable time of the crossover of HIV from chimpanzees into humans was earlier than 1957 to 1959, when the polio vaccine was used in the Congo.

However, according to Albert Sabin in a *British Medical Journal* article in 1959, he had discovered an "unidentified cell-killing virus" in Dr. Koprowski's vaccine. The year 1959 was also when the first known case of AIDS appeared in the Belgian Congo. Within the next few years, more cases of AIDS appeared in the areas where the Koprowski mass vaccination campaign had been conducted.

Although the use of contaminated polio vaccine may explain how HIV/AIDS began in Africa, why did it appear in dramatic numbers among homosexual men in North America? This was puzzling until 1992, when it was noted that beginning in the late 1970s, oral polio vaccines were often given to homosexual men as treatment for genital herpes. The treatments consisted of vaccines that were much more potent than those used to prevent polio. Because it is known that the polio viruses in the oral vaccine remain contagious in the stool, the sexual behaviors of homosexual men provide a logical way to transmit the disease.

In September 2000, the Royal Society in London met to discuss the origins of the HIV/AIDS epidemic. At the meeting, three independent laboratories selected by AIDS researchers gave the results of their investigations into samples of the original polio vaccines that are stored at the Wistar Institute in Philadelphia where the vaccines were developed. They reported that "there is nothing in the results from these tests to support the theory that HIV entered the human population during the late 1950s polio virus clinical trials in Africa." The laboratories also reported that there was no trace of chimpanzee DNA in the vaccine samples or any evidence of SIV or HIV in the samples.

Nevertheless there is still much we do not understand about

HIV/AIDS. While continuing investigations into the origins of the disease may not help those who already have HIV/AIDS, they could prevent similar problems of contamination in the future.

POLIO VACCINE AND CANCER

One of the little-known facts about the early polio vaccine is that millions of doses were contaminated with a monkey virus (SV40) that causes cancer in laboratory animals, but which government officials insist to this day is not dangerous to humans. Not everyone agrees with that claim, however.

SV40 appears to also have been involved in causing or contributing to a type of lung cancer called mesothelioma. The contaminated polio vaccine was administered to ninety-eight million Americans before the Food and Drug Administration required manufacturers to screen for the virus.

Despite the government's claim that SV40 is not linked to cancer, an independent study conducted at Loyola University in Chicago by Dr. Michele Carbone finds that "clearly, it is a risk factor in developing this disease." Dr. Carbone made this statement after finding SV40 in mesothelioma, which had previously been associated only with exposure to asbestos. Dr. Carbone found SV40 in 60 percent of the human mesotheliomas he studied.

Dr. Joseph R. Testa, a molecular geneticist and senior member of the Fox Chase Cancer Center in Philadelphia, directed Dr. Carbone's four-laboratory study in which each laboratory independently verified the findings of the others. He believes that government researchers should take a serious look at their findings. The National Cancer Institute (NCI) initiated a study of mesothelioma, which was overseen by Dr. Howard Strickler, an NCI epidemiologist. Barbara Loe Fisher questioned why the NCI study was not being monitored by a nongovernment molecular biologist. She believes that vaccine manufacturers and the government are afraid they will have a tremendous financial liability if it is found that millions of people were injected with a government-mandated vaccine that contains a cancer-causing monkey virus. Results of the NCI study are forthcoming.

Nearly three thousand people die of mesothelioma every year in the United States. Even though asbestos exposure is traditionally viewed as the cause of the disease, between 20 and 50 percent of cases involve people who have not been exposed to asbestos. The presence of SV40 may be a missing link.

But SV40 has been found in other cancers as well, including brain and bone cancers in children who never received the contaminated vaccine. This has led Dr. Carbone and others to speculate that the virus may be transmitted in utero from mother to child, in blood transfusions, or from sexual contact.

Cecil Fox, a senior scientist with the National Institutes of Health from 1973 until 1991, believes that the SV40 contamination problem highlights the risks of transmitting animal viruses when working with animal tissue. "When you inject ground-up monkey guts into children, all kinds of things can happen," he says.

BOTTOM LINE

The day may come when the polio vaccine is removed from the list of mandated vaccines for children. Certainly the virtual removal of the oral form is a big step in that direction. However, many questions about the polio vaccine still remain: Why are we still giving it even though the disease has been eliminated in the Western Hemisphere for more than two decades? Is there a link between the early contaminated polio vaccine and the origin of HIV/AIDS? Could a monkey virus that contaminated the polio vaccine forty-five years ago be causing some types of cancer today? And are the polio vaccines being given today still contaminated with monkey viruses?

Cecil Fox believes that monkey tissue will continue to be used because there is no financial incentive for vaccine makers to make a change.

Until the polio vaccine is no longer mandated, you can help protect your child by following the guidelines, "Actions Parents Can Take," in chapter 21, and by carefully considering the list of who should not get the polio vaccine.

NOTES

Bookchin, Debbie, and Jim Schumacher. "A New Cancer Risk?" *Newsday*, December 29, 1998.

Boston Magazine. "The Lonely Crusade of Walter Kyle." (June 1997).

Butel, J. S., and J. A. Lednicky. "Cell and Molecular Biology of Simian Virus 40: Implications for Human Infections and Disease." *Journal of the National Cancer Institute* 91, no. 2 (January 20, 1999): 119–34.

Centers for Disease Control and Prevention. Vaccine Information Statements. May 4, 2000.

Diodati, Catherine. *Immunization: History, Ethics, Law and Health.* Ontario, Canada: Integral Aspects, 1999, 8ff., 72, 114–20.

Fisher, Barbara Loe. *The Consumer's Guide to Childhood Vaccines.* Vienna, VA: National Vaccine Information Center, 1997.

Fisher, S. G., L. Weber, and M. Carbone. "Cancer Risk Associated with Simian Virus 40 Contaminated Polio Vaccine." *Anticancer Research* 19, no. 3B (May–June 1999): 2173–80.

Hirvonen, A., et al. "Simian Virus 40 (SV40)-Like DNA Sequences

Not Detectable in Finnish Mesothelioma Patients Not Exposed to SV40-Contaminated Polio Vaccines." *Molecular Carcinogens* 26, no. 2 (October 1999): 93–99.

Hoff, Brent, and Carter Smith. *Mapping Epidemics.* New York: Franklin Watts, 2000.

Horton, Richard. "New Data Challenge: OV Theory of AIDS Origin." *Lancet* 356: 1005.

Humiston, Sharon G., and Cynthia Good. *Vaccinating Your Child: Questions and Answers for the Concerned Parent.* Atlanta: Peachtree Publishers, 2000, 89–99.

The Institute for Vaccine Safety Web site: www.vaccinesafety.edu.

Kyle, W. "Simian Retroviruses, Polio Vaccine, and Origin of AIDS." *Lancet* 339 (1992).

Mendelsohn, Robert. *How to Raise a Healthy Child . . . In Spite of Your Doctor.* Chicago: Contemporary Books, 1984.

Miller, Neil Z. *Vaccine Safety Manual for Concerned Families and Health Practitioners.* Santa Fe: New Atlantean Press, 2008.

Neustaedter, Randall. *The Vaccine Guide: Making an Informed Choice.* Berkeley, CA: North Atlantic Books, 1996.

Chapter 10

❀

MMR: Measles, Mumps, Rubella

Measles, mumps, and rubella (German measles): three common childhood diseases that today's young parents likely never had as children. But baby boomers and pre-boomers know them well. Up through the mid-1960s, more than 90 percent of the US population caught measles by the time they were fifteen years old. During the 1964–65 outbreak of rubella, 12.5 million Americans had the disease. Mumps, although not as common as either of these other two diseases, still affected an estimated two hundred thousand people a year up until the late 1960s.

Today these diseases have nearly been eliminated in the United States, although they are still a significant problem in many parts of the developing world. Introduction of separate vaccines for each of the three infections during the 1960s, and recommendation of the combination vaccine (MMR) in 1979, contributed to a decrease in the incidence of the diseases.

But victories do not come without paying a price, and the MMR vaccine may be demanding payment. Ever since the early 1980s, the MMR vaccine has been a topic of controversy, as some parents have claimed that it is associated with autism and other neurological problems in their young children. That controversy continues today, and in fact is even more heated than it was in the beginning.

This chapter discusses measles, mumps, and rubella and then explores the three vaccines—and the combination vaccine—developed to prevent these infections. Central to the chapter is the continuing controversy around the safety of the MMR vaccine, and each of its components separately, including the serious adverse effects such as autism and autoimmune diseases linked with the vaccine.

MEASLES

Measles, also known as rubeola (not to be confused with rubella, which is explained below), is a highly contagious viral disease. Up until the late 1970s, it was one of the most common childhood diseases in the United States. Although nearly every child had had a bout with measles, the vast majority of them had no complications from the experience.

The measles virus is spread in the air in droplets that are released from infected people when they sneeze, cough, or talk. Other people can inhale the droplets, or the droplets can be deposited on surfaces or objects, such as utensils or toys, that children place in their mouths. The virus can remain contagious for two hours on such surfaces.

Who Gets Measles?

People of any age can get measles, although it is not common among children younger than six months or in adults twenty years and older. Today measles is nearly gone in the United States. However, the vast majority of the cases that do occur are among people who have been immunized. Some cases occur in Americans who have traveled abroad and brought it back with them, or from foreign visitors or immigrants who bring it with them.

In 1999, a record low of one hundred cases and no deaths were reported. In the years 1989 through 1991, however, there was an outbreak of measles that affected 53,632 people and caused 123 deaths. This outbreak apparently occurred when the first generation of measles-vaccinated mothers gave birth to babies. These babies did not have the protection of maternal antibodies that can be transferred to babies whose mothers have naturally recovered from the disease. Maternal antibodies protect babies for the first twelve to fifteen months of life. In the 1989–1991 measles outbreak, the majority of babies who died were under twelve months old and too young to be vaccinated— and in fact a number of older children who got measles had been vaccinated. There were also a number of inner-city children who had not been vaccinated.

Although the number of cases of measles has dropped dramatically, the age of people getting the disease has changed since introduction of the measles vaccine. In the pre-vaccine days, the average age of infections was four to five years. Today children aged ten to fourteen are most affected, followed by those five to nine years old and then fifteen to nineteen. It is believed the vaccine has pushed the disease into these older age groups and that one measles shot does not confer lifelong immunity, so the CDC now recommends a second dose.

Symptoms and Treatment

About four days before and up to six days after symptoms appear, a person with measles is contagious. The first symptoms to appear are a hacking cough, fatigue, sore throat, runny nose, conjunctivitis (redness and inflammation of the inner eyelids), and fever. The conjunctivitis may be accompanied by discharge. Often the back of the throat is very red and the tongue and tonsils have a yellow coating. About four days after these symptoms appear, a red, bumpy rash begins, usually on the neck and face. The rash gradually spreads to the trunk, arms, and legs over the next few days as it fades from the face. Sometimes the bumps form large, blotchy areas.

Among people who get measles beyond age five or those who get the disease despite having been immunized, there have been reports of unusual forms of the disease, which suggests that the virus is mutating. Some of those symptoms include an abnormal rash, persistent high fever, hypoxia (lack of oxygen in the cells, which affects the heart and respiration), and pneumonia.

Treatment of measles includes controlling fever with acetaminophen and baths if needed. The cough should not be suppressed, but placing a humidifier in the room can be helpful. The diet should contain plenty of fruits and vegetables, especially those high in vitamin A (for example, carrots, cantaloupe, yellow squash, yellow peppers), and drinking lots of fluids is encouraged.

Complications of Measles

If a pregnant woman gets measles, there is a risk of premature birth, low birth weight, and infant death. Scientists do not know if measles during pregnancy causes birth defects. However, there is evidence that some women who get the measles vaccine (including MMR) before or during pregnancy give birth to children who develop autism or other neurological or behavioral problems, and that women who get the vaccine after giving birth and who then breast-feed have children who can develop the same problems. (See chapter 4 for a discussion of the link between MMR and autism.)

Between 6 and 8 percent of people who get measles also get pneumonia, ear infection, or diarrhea. In rare cases (1 out of 1,000), the measles virus affects the brain and causes inflammation (encephalitis). Symptoms of encephalitis usually include convulsions, confusion, and sometimes coma. One out of 1,000 people with measles die.

MUMPS

Mumps, like measles, is a viral disease that usually occurs in childhood and early adolescence. Although it is spread like measles—through the air on droplets released from infected people when they sneeze, talk, or cough—it is not as contagious as measles.

Who Gets Mumps?

Mumps is most common in children five to nineteen years old. In 1964, there were an estimated 212,000 cases of mumps in the United States. Since the introduction of the vaccine, the number of cases has dropped to about 387 per year (in 1999).

Symptoms and Treatment

The mumps virus can cause inflammation in various parts of the body. The area most often affected, and the most obvious, is the salivary gland (parotid gland) in the mouth, which causes the cheeks to puff out. The virus may also attack the pancreas, ovaries, testes, and, in rare cases, the meninges (tissue that lines the brain). Other common symptoms include fever and fatigue.

If a child develops meningitis (inflammation of the meninges), symptoms include a headache and a stiff neck. Signs that the mumps virus has attacked the pancreas include pain in the upper part of the belly, while some people also experience nausea and vomiting. Females whose ovaries are affected normally feel pain in the lower abdomen.

In about 25 percent of males who get mumps, the virus also affects one or both testes. This condition, known as orchitis, causes the testis to be painful and tender for two to four days. The affected testis may shrink. In extremely rare cases, the inflammation in the testis can damage the sperm and cause sterility. Men who had mumps as children can undergo a semen analysis to determine if their sperm is still viable.

Treatment of mumps includes acetaminophen for fever and pain, ice or heat on the swollen neck and face, and saltwater gargles for the throat. Children should not take aspirin because of the risk of Reye's syndrome.

RUBELLA (GERMAN MEASLES)

Rubella, or German measles, is a viral disease that spreads in the same way as measles. Many people who get rubella do not have symptoms, but they can still spread the disease.

Rubella was once a very common childhood illness in the

United States. During the 1964–65 outbreak, 12.5 million Americans had the disease. Although rubella is generally a mild disease for most people, it can be fatal or very damaging to a fetus. Among the 12.5 million Americans who had rubella during the 1964–65 outbreak were many pregnant women; about 11,000 had spontaneous or therapeutic abortions, and another 20,000 infants were born with disabilities, including mental retardation, deafness, and blindness. These young victims of their mothers' rubella had what is known as congenital rubella syndrome (CRS; see below).

Outbreaks of rubella among unvaccinated adults resulted in more than one thousand cases in 1990 and 1991. Since 1992, cases of rubella and CRS have remained relatively low (rubella: 128 cases in 1995, 213 in 1996, and 364 in 1998; CRS, 4 cases in 1995, 2 in 1996, and 7 in 1998). However, because reporting of CRS is voluntary in the United States, it is believed that the reported totals are only 40 to 70 percent of the actual total.

Who Gets Rubella?

Before the rubella vaccine became available in 1969 (it was developed in 1966), preschool- and elementary-school-aged children were the ones who most often got the disease. But since the vaccine has been widely used, people in their twenties and thirties are getting the disease, even though the total number of cases has dropped dramatically. In 1997 in the United States, 161 people caught rubella, and 75 percent of them were between the ages of twenty and thirty-nine. And as is explained below, rubella is more serious in adults.

Symptoms and Treatment

Rubella often does not cause symptoms. When it does, young children usually get a rash while adolescents and adults typically develop symptoms of a common cold, swollen glands, and then a rash.

Among adults who get rubella, arthritis is a common complication, especially among women. Encephalitis occurs in about 1 out of every 6,000 cases and affects adults more than it does children, while thrombocytopenia (reduced levels of platelets) is seen more often in children and in 1 out of every 3,000 cases.

Pregnancy and Complications of Rubella

While rubella itself does not cause serious symptoms in most people, it can be devastating when it is contracted by pregnant women. When rubella occurs during early pregnancy, the result is often congenital rubella syndrome, which includes miscarriage, stillbirths, fetal anomalies (for example, deafness, cataracts, glaucoma, heart defects, mental retardation, bone defects, and poor growth), and therapeutic abortions.

Congenital rubella syndrome has been estimated to affect 20 to 25 percent of infants born to women who acquire rubella during their first twenty weeks of pregnancy, but some believe this figure is low. In fact, some studies show that 85 percent of infants born to mothers who were infected during the first eight weeks of pregnancy had CRS. The risk of CRS decreases as the pregnancy advances, and women who are infected after the twentieth week rarely give birth to an infant with CRS. During the last rubella epidemic in the United States (1964–65), before the vaccine became available, there were an estimated twenty thousand cases of CRS.

THE MMR VACCINE

The MMR vaccine was not born as a trio: Each vaccine was developed independently (measles 1963; rubella 1966; mumps 1968), then they were combined into MMR and recommended for use in 1979. That does not mean your child must get the combination vaccine. You can request that he or she get a separate vaccine for each of these diseases (see "Actions Parents Can Take" in chapter 21).

Measles Vaccine

The quest for a measles vaccine began in earnest in 1911, when Joseph Goldberger and John Anderson discovered that the disease was caused by a virus. They found that monkeys could be infected with measles, which gave them a model in which to test the vaccine. The first vaccine in humans was tested on military recruits in 1940, but it caused such severe reactions that it was withdrawn. Two other vaccines were introduced in 1963–64, a live and an inactivated form. The inactivated vaccine proved to cause measles. The live, attenuated measles vaccine used today (Enders-Edmonston strain) was licensed in 1968 and is the only measles virus vaccine available in the United States. By the late 1960s, the live vaccine was in use.

The measles vaccine is available alone, in the MMR combination, and in a measles-rubella form. All forms contain the antibiotic neomycin and the stabilizers sorbitol and gelatin. The measles virus is grown in chick embryo cell culture.

How Effecive Is the Measles Vaccine?

In 1989, the CDC reported measles outbreaks in schools in which 98 to 100 percent of the children had been vaccinated. These occurrences led experts with the Mayo Vaccine Research Group to say that "the apparent paradox is that as measles immunization rates rise to high levels in a population, measles becomes a disease of immunized persons." There is also some concern that measles vaccination suppresses the immune system and can lead to an increased susceptibility to other infections, as reported by Dr. P. G. Auwaeter and his colleagues in their research in 1996.

There is evidence that the measles virus may be growing resistant to the vaccines. The CDC has identified eight different genotypes of wild measles virus throughout the world that may have occurred because the vaccine has forced the virus to mutate. The CDC also has reported a 1998 measles outbreak in Alaska in which 51 percent of the children who got the measles had received at least one of the two recommended doses of measles vaccine.

Mumps Vaccine

Even though the live mumps vaccine was available in 1968, it was not used routinely before 1977. Before the vaccine was introduced, children five to nine years were the most likely to get the disease. Thus, most people born before 1957 were probably infected naturally between 1957 and 1977 and presumed to be immune. However, being born before 1957 does not guarantee immunity to mumps. Therefore the CDC recommends that during a mumps outbreak, the MMR vaccine should be considered for anyone born before 1957 who may be exposed to the disease.

The only mumps vaccine available now in the United States is a live virus vaccine that is grown in cell cultures of chick embryo. The mumps vaccine is available alone, in the MMR combination, and in a rubella-mumps combination. Each form contains the live attenuated virus plus human albumin (a protein found in blood that is added to vaccines as a stabilizer), the antibiotic neomycin, and the stabilizers sorbitol and gelatin.

How Effective Is the Mumps Vaccine?

More than 97 percent of people who are susceptible to mumps develop measurable levels of antibodies to the disease. However, field studies show that the vaccine is only 75 to 95 percent effective. It is unknown exactly how long vaccine-induced immunity lasts, but data gathered over the years since the vaccine was first administered indicate that it is good for at least thirty years.

Several studies show an increase in the number of mumps cases soon after required mumps immunization began. One study looked at an outbreak in 1991 in Tennessee among junior high and high school students. Of the sixty-eight cases of mumps that occurred, sixty-seven children had been vaccinated. Before the mumps vaccine became mandatory in the school in 1988, mumps had been uncommon in the area. In fact, from 1971 through 1979, there were only eighty-five cases, and none had been reported in the 1980s. A mumps outbreak in 2007 in eight Midwestern states raised questions about the effectiveness of the MMR vaccine routinely given to children. More than six hundred cases were reported in Iowa compared with three the previous year. Sixty-four percent of the children in Iowa who came down with the disease had two doses of the MMR vaccine. An additional 10 percent had one dose.

A CDC representative said that the vaccine is working. The

CDC reports the vaccine is 90 to 95 percent effective and that immunity should last more than twenty-five years. A possible explanation was gleaned from a study by Robert M. Jacobson in the Department of Pediatrics and Adolescent Medicine, Mayo Clinic, Rochester, Minnesota. He discovered that a genetic phenomenon explains the measles vaccine failure, which is no more than 0.2 percent. He found groups of children clustered in families who demonstrated a failed antibody response after the vaccine was given. Possibly the same happens with the mumps vaccine.

Who Really Needs the Mumps Vaccine?

The mumps vaccine was apparently developed to protect adult males who do not get the disease during childhood—and thus acquire natural immunity—to avoid the rare possibility that they would become sterile. The risk of sterility is actually very low among males who get mumps, especially since if the virus does affect the testes, it usually affects only one, leaving the other one viable.

If the mumps vaccine was developed for males, why are females also immunized? As with the immunization of children for rubella, which is described below under "Rubella Vaccine: Should We Immunize Children," giving the mumps vaccine to girls places one population at risk of adverse reactions and complications for the sake of another. In this case, immunizing girls reduces the chance that they will expose males to the disease.

Another problem with the mumps vaccine is that since it was introduced, the number of mumps cases has declined among young children (preadolescent) and increased among adolescents and adults. This is a significant problem because, like measles and rubella, mumps causes much more serious complications among older people than among children.

Rubella Vaccine

The rubella vaccine is available alone or in the MMR combination, in a measles-rubella combination, and in a rubella-mumps combination. Each dose of these vaccines contains the antibiotic neomycin, along with sorbitol and gelatin as stabilizers. The live rubella vaccine is grown in a culture of human cells taken from a fetus aborted in 1964 after the mother got rubella.

Rubella Vaccine: Should We Immunize Children?

Beginning in 1969, mass immunization for rubella was targeted at young children: The CDC hoped to interrupt the spread of the virus and eliminate the risk of exposure among pregnant women because of the risk of CRS. This vaccination approach is what Catherine Diodati describes in her book *Immunization: History, Ethics, Law and Health* as a clear example of "immunization for utilitarian purposes." That means it was designed to protect not the recipient of the vaccine, but another population: in this case, the fetuses of susceptible pregnant women. In fact, this population is the only group really at risk for the disease. For all others, according to researcher Jean H. Joncas, "Rubella is . . . a benign disease that does not justify prevention by vaccination."

Some experts believe that immunizing young children for rubella is not justified, and they also note that it places them at risk of adverse reactions, including arthritis, autism, and behavioral disorders (see chapters 4 and 5).

Another phenomenon associated with this vaccination approach has occurred. Between 1969 and 1976 the number of reported cases of rubella decreased from 57,600 to 12,400. Although this was good, a closer look shows a disturbing trend. Whereas young children made up more than 75 percent of cases before 1969, by 1975 through 1977, people aged fifteen years and older made up 62 percent of those with the disease, compared with only 23 percent of the cases in earlier years.

This was not good, because now those most likely to have complications—pregnant women—were getting the disease. Dr. J. D. Cherry, a member of the Advisory Committee on Immunization Practices, noted in 1980 that "essentially we have controlled the disease in persons 14 years of age or younger but have given it a free hand in those 15 or older."

Experts who question mass vaccination for rubella note that the disease is mild in children and that the naturally acquired disease produces immunity in at least 80 percent of people. This means that only a small percentage of people would need immunization later on in life, rather than injecting all children and exposing them to pain, discomfort, and the risk of adverse reactions.

The MMR Vaccine

The MMR vaccine contains the three live attenuated viruses plus human albumin, the antibiotic neomycin, and the stabilizers sorbitol and gelatin. There is no preservative. It is injected just under the skin.

KATHY'S STORY

At fifteen months, Kathy had already been walking for two months and was a healthy, happy toddler. Her mother dutifully brought her in for her first MMR vaccine, and nine days later she noted that Kathy had a low-grade fever and a runny nose. Because her doctor had warned her that cold-like symptoms could occur, Kathy's mother did not worry. However, as the cold symptoms disappeared, so did her daughter's cheerful, playful disposition. When Kathy began to trip and fall down a lot, the doctor told her mother to put ice on the vaccine injection site and to give her acetaminophen.

But instead of improving, Kathy got worse. She lost her ability to walk or sit and became paralyzed from the waist down. Suspicions of a spinal cord tumor proved to be negative, but a brain scan showed white lesions on her brain, indicating brain damage. She would have a fever for several days nearly every week, yet repeated lab tests showed nothing unusual.

With the help of steroid therapy, doctors were able to stop Kathy's brain from deteriorating further. Her parents filed for compensation under the Vaccine Injury Compensation Program and won their claim in 1993 after a US Court of Claims ruled that Kathy had encephalopathy (brain inflammation and damage) as a result of her MMR vaccination. Kathy is confined to a wheelchair.

Adverse Reactions to MMR: The CDC

According to the Vaccine Information Statements issued by the CDC, most people who get the MMR vaccine do not have any side effects. They also state that getting the vaccine is much safer than getting any of the diseases it is designed to prevent. The next few pages list the side effects associated with the vaccine.

Mild

If these adverse effects occur, they usually happen within seven to twelve days after receiving the shot. They are less likely to occur after receiving the second dose.

- Fever: up to 1 person out of 6.
- Mild rash: about 1 person out of 20.
- Swollen glands in the neck or cheeks: rare.

Moderate

- Seizure caused by fever: about 1 out of 3,000 doses.
- Pain and stiffness in the joints (temporary), usually seen in teenage or adult women: up to 1 out of 4.
- Low platelet count (thrombocytopenia; temporary), which can cause a bleeding disorder: about 1 out of 30,000 doses.

Severe

The CDC says that severe reactions to MMR are very rare. They include:

- Serious allergic reactions that include difficulty breathing, hives, weakness, paleness, fast heartbeat, dizziness, and wheezing or hoarseness: less than 1 out of 1 million doses.
- Other reactions that the CDC says have been known to occur but cannot be linked with the vaccine include long-term seizures, coma, reduced consciousness, permanent brain damage, and deafness.

Other Adverse Reactions

The National Vaccine Information Center notes that in addition to the adverse reactions cited by the CDC, other events have been reported. These include stinging and burning at the injection site, sore throat, cough, headache, nausea and vomiting, diarrhea, ear infections, conjunctivitis, retinitis, arthritis, Guillain-Barré syndrome (progressive muscle weakness), encephalopathy (degenerative brain disease), and subacute sclerosing panencephalitis (a rare, fatal brain disease). There is also a continuing debate over whether MMR causes Crohn's disease and other gastrointestinal (GI) tract diseases, including inflammatory bowel disease and colitis. The key researcher in this area is Andrew Wakefield, M.D., a London pediatric gastroenterologist. His findings are discussed in chapter 5.

Reports of adverse reactions associated with the MMR vaccine have been the center of a growing controversy ever since the early 1980s when parents reported that the vaccine appeared to be linked with autism and other neurological problems in their children. The body of evidence to support these claims is growing (see chapter 4).

FEDERAL/STATE GUIDELINES FOR MMR DOSING

According to the CDC, children should get two doses of MMR vaccine based on the following schedule:

- First dose at twelve to fifteen months of age.
- Second dose at four to six years of age.

Although this is the recommended dosing schedule, children can get their second dose at any age if they receive it at least twenty-eight days after the first dose. The CDC also recommends that anyone eighteen years of age or older who was born after 1956 should get at least one dose of MMR unless they have had a dose of the vaccine or have had the diseases. Adults who travel abroad, go to college, or work in the health care field may need to get an MMR shot. As a way to avoid the shot, you can get a blood test to check your antibody levels for these diseases before getting the vaccine.

Who Should Not Get the MMR Vaccine?

The CDC recommends that individuals who fit into the following categories should not get the MMR vaccine or should wait:

- Anyone who has ever had a life-threatening allergic reaction to gelatin, the antibiotic neomycin, or to a previous MMR shot.
- People who are moderately or seriously ill at the time the shot is scheduled should wait until they have recovered before getting the vaccine. (For another opinion, see "Actions Parents Can Take" in chapter 21.)
- Pregnant women should wait until they have given birth to get the MMR vaccine. If a woman gets an MMR vaccine, she should not get pregnant for at least three months. Although the CDC does not mention guidelines for breast-feeding women, some experts believe the vaccine can be passed to infants through breast milk and so recommend that breast-feeding women not get the vaccine.

- People in the following situations similarly should check with their doctor before getting the MMR vaccine: women who are breast-feeding; anyone with HIV/AIDS, an immune system disease (for example, chronic fatigue syndrome or lupus), cancer, or a low platelet count; anyone who is receiving cancer treatment; people who have been taking medications that affect the immune system (for example, steroids) for two weeks or longer; and people who have recently had a blood transfusion or who have received blood products.

SERIOUS REACTIONS: WHAT TO LOOK FOR, WHAT TO DO

According to the CDC, moderate or severe reactions to MMR vaccine should be reported to and checked by a doctor immediately. Most of the reactions listed here (except for high fever, seizure, brain damage, and behavior changes), if they were to occur, would happen within a few minutes to a few hours after the shot. The CDC states that permanent brain damage and deafness have been known to occur after MMR vaccinations, but that it is not clear if the vaccine was the cause. If a high fever or seizure were to occur, it would happen one to two weeks after the shot. All adverse reactions should also be reported to the Vaccine Adverse Events Reporting System (VAERS), which is explained in chapter 22. Signs to look for include:

- Behavior changes
- Difficulty breathing
- Hoarseness or wheezing

- Weakness
- Fast heartbeat
- Dizziness
- Hives
- Paleness
- High fever
- Seizure
- Permanent brain damage or deafness

BOTTOM LINE

Before you take your child in for his or her MMR vaccine, carefully review the list of "Who Should Not Get the MMR Vaccine?" in this chapter. If your child does not fit into any of those categories and you still wish to proceed, I feel that it is safer for children to get the individual components of the vaccine six months apart, starting with the measles shot first at fifteen months, followed by rubella six months later, and by mumps six months after the rubella shot. Monitor your child after each dose, record any adverse reactions, and consult with your doctor about whether subsequent doses should be given. Check your child's titers at four to five years of age to see if he or she needs a booster. Also, follow the suggestions listed at the end of chapter 21 to help protect your child against possible reactions to the vaccines. I generally recommend that if pregnant women are found to be negative when tested for immunity to rubella, they should only be vaccinated with rubella at the proper time (after birth and breast-feeding), not with the MMR.

In the event that the separate vaccines are unavailable, refer to chapter 21.

NOTES

Auwaeter, P. G., et al. "Changes Within T Cell Receptor V-beta Subsets in Infants Following Measles Vaccination." *Clinical Immunology Immunopathology* 79, no. 2 (May 1996): 163–70.

Centers for Disease Control and Prevention. Vaccine Information Statements. May 4, 2000.

———. "Measles." *Morbidity and Mortality Weekly* 38 (1989): 329–30; and 33 (1984).

Centers for Disease Control and Prevention Web site: www.cdc.org.

CureResearch.com Web site: www.cureresearch.com.

Diodati, Catherine. *Immunization: History, Ethics, Law and Health.* Ontario, Canada: Integral Aspects, 1999, 17, 108–10.

Fisher, Barbara Loe. *The Consumer's Guide to Childhood Vaccines.* Vienna, VA: National Vaccine Information Center, 1997.

Joncas, Jean H. "Preventing the Congenital Rubella Syndrome by Vaccinating Women at Risk." *Canadian Medical Association Journal* 129, no. 2 (July 15, 1983): 110.

Koch, Kathy. "Vaccine Controversies." *CQ Researcher* (August 2000): 650.

Mayo Vaccine Research Group. "Failure to Reach the Goal of Measles Elimination: Apparent Paradox of Measles Infections in Unimmunized Persons." *Archives of Internal Medicine* 154, no. 16 (August 22, 1994): 1815–20.

Nussinovitch, M., et al. "Arthritis After Mumps and Measles Vaccination." *Archives of Disease in Childhood* 72 (1995): 348–49.

Scheibner, Viera. *Vaccination: 100 Years of Orthodox Research Shows That Vaccines Represent a Medical Assault on the Immune System,* citing Cherry, 111.

Chapter 11

❋

Varicella (Chicken Pox)

As diseases go, chicken pox (also called varicella) is a relatively mild one, especially when you compare it with the often deadly illnesses for which some other vaccines have been developed. True, chicken pox can be especially dangerous for children who have a weakened immune system, such as those who have leukemia or other cancers, which puts them at high risk of complications from chicken pox. In fact, that is one of the reasons the varicella vaccine was developed: to reduce the complications, including death, that are possible in this small but vulnerable population of children.

But there appears to be another reason the varicella vaccine was developed, one that has little to do with helping this select group of children. The reason is that the government was looking for a way to save businesses hundreds of millions of dollars in lost production time, because working mothers had to stay home when their children got sick. The solution: develop a vaccine for chicken pox so moms could keep working instead of taking time off to nurse their kids. The savings, calculated by Merck

Laboratories, the makers of the only chicken pox vaccine on the market, were estimated to be $400 million.

Apparently marketing the vaccine to every child in the United States does have a cost benefit. So the bottom line is that Americans have yet another vaccine mandated in many states as a requirement for children to get into school. And like other vaccines, it has its share of fans and opponents and a list of unique and troublesome characteristics. To help you learn all you can about this vaccine before you decide if you or your children should or should not be vaccinated, this chapter explores the varicella vaccine and the disease it was designed to prevent.

CHICKEN POX

Chicken pox, or varicella, is a common childhood disease caused by the varicella zoster virus. Without vaccination, between 85 and 90 percent of people will get chicken pox. The chicken pox virus spreads from person to person in the airborne droplets sprayed into the air through coughing, speaking, and sneezing, or by contact with fluid from the blisters that appear on the skin as part of the disease. It can also be caught from people who have shingles, which is a complication of chicken pox. Once people are exposed to the chicken pox virus, it takes two to three weeks for symptoms, including rash, to appear.

How Common Is Chicken Pox?

In 1992, about 158,000 cases of chicken pox and 100 related deaths, mostly in adults, were reported in the United States. Yet the CDC believes this is only the tip of the iceberg. The agency states that an estimated 4 to 5 percent of the approximately 3.7 million cases of the disease are reported each year. The reason for the huge difference between the reported and estimated actual numbers is that reporting by the states has been poor, with only about fourteen states reporting cases at all, and their figures are not always complete. This lack of uniform reporting has made it difficult to monitor the impact of the varicella vaccine on the disease. It is estimated that there has been a 90 percent decline in reported cases and a 66 percent decline in deaths following the introduction of the vaccine.

Who Gets Chicken Pox?

About 50 percent of all cases of chicken pox in the United States occur in children between the ages of five and nine, with fewer cases found in younger children. The vast majority of children who get chicken pox recover completely in two to three weeks and have permanent immunity to the disease. Among children who have weakened immune systems, such as those with leukemia or other forms of cancer, a thousand or more lesions may erupt on their skin. Some of these children then develop complications, including brain inflammation and death.

When chicken pox occurs in adolescents or adults, which it is doing with increasing frequency for reasons explained below, the consequences can be serious. Up to 20 percent of adults who get chicken pox also get pneumonia accompanied by chest pain, fever, persistent cough, and inflamed lungs. Some adults develop liver and heart problems, lesions on their cornea, and arthritis. The death rate among adults who get chicken pox is 31 per 100,000 cases.

Pregnant women who get chicken pox during their first or early second trimester risk giving birth to a child with birth defects. To prevent chicken pox during pregnancy, the CDC recommends that women make sure they are immune before they get pregnant.

Symptoms and Treatment

The first symptoms of chicken pox are a low-grade fever and fatigue, followed in a day or two by an itchy rash. The lesions, or pox, usually first appear on the back, face, and chest and then spread rapidly over the entire body. At first the lesions look like pimples, but then they transform into blisters that contain a contagious fluid. The number of lesions can range from less than ten to hundreds. Generally, younger children have fewer lesions than do older children or adults, and the more lesions are present, the higher the fever.

To help reduce the itching, tepid-water baths, soaking in a baking soda or oatmeal bath, and wet, cool compresses offer some relief. Aspirin should not be given to reduce fever, because its use during chicken pox can cause a potentially fatal disease called Reye's syndrome, which affects the brain and liver. To prevent children from scratching the lesions, cut their nails short. Scratching the lesions can cause them to become infected with bacteria, which can lead to scars, tissue damage, or, in rare cases, death.

Shingles: A Later-Life Complication

After individuals recover from chicken pox, the virus doesn't go away. Instead it lives quietly in the nerve cells near the base of the spine. Then it can erupt into a condition known as shingles. This is a condition in which the revitalized chicken pox virus causes painful, often burning blisters on the skin. Because these blisters contain the chicken pox virus, people with shingles are contagious and can transmit chicken pox to susceptible individuals.

Shingles most often occurs in people aged fifty years and older because immunity to the varicella zoster virus decreases as people age. Americans have a one in five chance of getting shingles during their lifetime, and they can get it more than once. Between six hundred thousand and a million Americans get shingles each year. Episodes are brought on by stress or other events that can weaken the immune system, such as a prolonged illness, cancer therapy, severe malnutrition, old age, or AIDS.

While in the past shingles has normally been seen in people over fifty, since the introduction of the varicella vaccine there have been reports of shingles in children. Some would argue that the vaccine has been associated with this pattern of earlier onset.

CHICKEN POX (VARICELLA) VACCINE

In 1972, a Japanese scientist named Michiaki Takahaski, M.D., isolated the chicken pox virus from the blood of a three-year-old Japanese boy. Dr. Takahaski then weakened (attenuated) the virus by growing it in various culture media, including human embryonic lung cell cultures and embryonic guinea pig cell cultures, and finally human diploid (two sets of chromosomes) cell cultures. The weakened virus was tested in children, and when it proved successful, the Merck pharmaceutical company bought the rights to use the strain—named Oka for the three-year-old boy—and began work to develop its own vaccine.

Unlike other attenuated viruses used to make vaccines (for example, polio and measles), in which the viruses emerge unaided from the cultivated cells, the chicken pox virus must be "broken out" of the cell. To do this, Merck uses ultrasound, which creates heat, which could damage the fragile varicella virus. To minimize problems, Merck uses robots to handle the virus and the vaccine-making process. That process includes the addition of sucrose, phosphate, glutamate, and gelatin to the vaccine to stabilize it.

In May 1993, Merck submitted the results of its safety and

effectiveness tests for the new vaccine, named Varivax, to the FDA. The FDA licensed Varivax in 1995, seven years after Japan and Korea had licensed a chicken pox vaccine.

How Effective Is the Vaccine?

The vaccine is estimated to be between 70 and 90 percent effective and to remain so for up to ten years after immunization. This is only an estimate, however. As stated in the manufacturer's product information, "The duration of protection is unknown at present and the need for booster doses is not defined." The vaccine is not effective in children younger than one year. Up to 5 percent of children do get a mild case of chicken pox, usually fewer than fifty pox, within a year or so of their vaccination.

FEDERAL/STATE GUIDELINES FOR VARICELLA VACCINE DOSING

The recommendation by the CDC in 2008 is for each child to receive two doses of the varicella vaccine at least three months apart if the child is under the age of thirteen and two doses of the vaccine at least four weeks apart if the child is thirteen or older.

I do not recommend that any child receive the varicella vaccine on the same day as the measles, mumps, or rubella vaccines or the MMR as a combination. Proquad was distributed by Merck as a combination vaccine for MMRV (measles, mumps, rubella, varicella). There was a move to discontinue this combination vaccine in 2008 because of the side effects encountered.

Who Should Not Get the Vaccine?

The CDC recommends that people who fall into any of the following categories should not get the vaccine, or should delay it:

- People who have a condition that compromises the immune system, including leukemia, other cancers, and HIV/AIDS; as well as those receiving drugs that affect the immune system, such as steroids, for two weeks or longer. People who are undergoing cancer treatment should consult their doctor to see if the varicella vaccine is safe for them.
- Pregnant women. Because contracting chicken pox during pregnancy may result in birth defects to the fetus, women who have not had the disease or who have not been vaccinated and wish to be immunized should wait until after the pregnancy is over. Women who want to be immunized before becoming pregnant should wait at least one month after receiving the vaccine to become pregnant to help ensure that the virus in the vaccine does not affect the fetus.
- Those with a moderate or severe illness.
- People who have ever had a life-threatening allergic reaction to the antibiotic neomycin or to gelatin (both used in the production of the vaccine), or to a previous dose of varicella vaccine (if a second dose is needed).
- Anyone who has recently had a blood transfusion or who has received other blood products should consult his or her doctor before getting the vaccine.

Adverse Reactions

According to the Vaccine Information Statement (VIS) issued by the CDC, most people who get chicken pox vaccine experience no side effects. The VIS reports the adverse effects to be as follows:

- Tenderness or swelling at the injection site: 1 child out of 5, and up to 1 out of 3 adolescents and adults.
- Fever: 1 out of 10 or fewer.
- Mild rash, which can appear up to one month after receiving the vaccine: 1 out of 20 or fewer. People with this rash can infect others.
- Seizures, caused by fever: 1 out of 1,000.
- Pneumonia.
- Other reactions, which reportedly are rare, include low blood count and severe brain reactions.

Adverse Effects: Another Look

On September 13, 2000, five years after the varicella vaccine was introduced to the US market, the Food and Drug Administration (FDA) reported to the American public that between March 1995 and July 1998 a total of 6,574 adverse events related to the vaccine had been reported to the Vaccine Adverse Events Reporting System (VAERS). This total represented 67.5 adverse reaction reports per 100,000 doses of the vaccine sold between those two dates. Included in these figures is the fact that approximately 4 percent (1 in 33,000 doses) of the reactions were serious and included shock, convulsions, thrombocytopenia, encephalitis, and fourteen deaths.

Although these numbers are serious, what the authors of the report stated is even more so: The 6,574 figure underreports the actual number of cases, a generally recognized fact in the medical community about other figures released from VAERS. In fact, it is believed that only 10 percent of all adverse events are reported to VAERS (see chapter 22). That means instead of 6,574 adverse events, the actual figure may be closer to 66,000.

Barbara Loe Fisher, president of the National Vaccine Information Center (NVIC), responded to the report by saying that "We have been getting reports from parents that their children are suffering high fevers, chicken pox lesions, shingles (Herpes zoster), brain damage and dying after chicken pox vaccination, especially when the vaccine is given at the same time with MMR and other vaccines. This FDA report confirms our concern that the chicken pox vaccine may be more reactive than anticipated in individuals with both known and unknown biological high risk factors."

Yet despite the 6,574 adverse effects and the admitted underreporting, the FDA labeled the vaccine's risks as "minimal." The NVIC's response to this conclusion was that it does "not match the substance of the data presented." Furthermore, the NVIC immediately called for further evaluation of the short- and long-term effects of the vaccine, especially among people with weakened immune systems, such as those with asthma or other chronic illnesses. The NVIC also wants doctors to stop giving the varicella vaccine simultaneously with other vaccines, especially MMR, because of the high number of adverse effects also seen with this vaccine.

Two children presented with signs of a stroke five days and three weeks after receiving the varicella vaccine. This happened at the Alberta Children's Hospital in Ontario, Canada, in 2004.

Testing the Vaccine

Before the FDA approved the varicella vaccine, Merck tested it on about eleven thousand children and adults. One of the concerns expressed by some experts was whether the vaccine would provide lifetime immunity or push the disease into adulthood (see "Shot Now, Pay Later," below). Philip Krause, M.D., a senior research investigator in the FDA's Center for Biologics Evaluation and Research, reported that over the five years the vaccine was studied the FDA did not see any evidence that immunity decreased. However, he also admitted that the FDA does not know how long beyond the five years immunity will last. "The only way to sort that out is going to be to see what happens after the vaccine is introduced," he said. The FDA asked Merck to follow several thousand vaccinated children for fifteen years to determine the long-term effects of the vaccine and to see if there would be a need for a booster shot. The preliminary results point to a conclusion that a booster is needed. At the present, the recommendation is for a primary vaccination and a booster.

A Few Words from the Manufacturer

Vaccine manufacturers often include information on their product inserts that does not appear on the Vaccine Information Statement given to parents. For the varicella vaccine, the following warnings come with the package:

- "Individuals vaccinated with [the vaccine] may potentially be capable of transmitting the vaccine virus to close contacts. Therefore, vaccine recipients should avoid close association with susceptible high risk individuals (e.g., newborns, pregnant women, immunocompromised persons)."
- "It is also not known whether [the vaccine] can cause fetal harm when administered to a pregnant woman or can affect reproduction capacity" and "it is not known whether Varicella vaccine virus is secreted in human milk. Therefore, because

some viruses are secreted in human milk, caution should be exercised if [the vaccine] is administered to a nursing woman."

- "[The vaccine] has not been evaluated for its carcinogenic or mutagenic potential, or its potential to impair fertility."

SHOT NOW, PAY LATER?
PUSHING CHICKEN POX INTO ADULTHOOD

One major concern that I share with many experts and parent groups is that mass immunization of young children with the varicella vaccine will force the disease to take hold in older individuals, in whom the disease often causes serious, even deadly, complications. This possibility is based on two factors: that immunity from the vaccine may wear off—which has already been determined by the manufacturer—and that the disease will not be as prevalent in the population as the years pass. These two factors work together in creating this concern.

It works like this: As more and more healthy children are vaccinated today, there will be a decreasing number of unvaccinated children who will have an opportunity to get chicken pox and acquire permanent natural immunity. When both the vaccinated and the unvaccinated children reach adulthood, many may be at risk for getting chicken pox and experiencing serious complications. If, however, children are allowed to get chicken pox (which is usually mild in childhood), they will have permanent immunity and thus eliminate the risk of getting the disease in adulthood.

Dr. Jane Seward, acting deputy director of the US Centers for Disease Control and Prevention's division of viral diseases, published a study looking at the length of protection against chicken pox in children vaccinated with the varicella vaccine in the March 15, 2008, issue of the *New England Journal of Medicine.* The study found the incidence of chicken pox among vaccinated children increasing over time from 1.6 cases per year one year after vaccination to 9 cases per year five years later, and more than 58 cases per year nine years later.

Shingles

The varicella vaccine also holds another possible risk. It's been shown that the vaccine can cause shingles in children, even though shingles nearly always occurs only in adults. In the *Journal of Infectious Diseases,* vaccine expert Stanley Plotkin reports that two children who received the varicella vaccine developed shingles four years after their vaccination. He also notes that in Japan, where the vaccine has been given for several years longer than in the United States, there have been many cases of shingles in children.

In the United States, however, the FDA gives conflicting statements about the possibility the vaccine may cause shingles in children or later in life. "Based on our knowledge of how the virus works and the data available so far, it doesn't appear that the rate of shingles cases in vaccinated individuals will be any greater than the naturally infected population," says Dr. Philip Krause of the FDA in an *FDA Consumer* article. Yet at the same time he admits, "Nobody's sure what the effect will be. We really don't have the data to say what's going to happen in twenty to thirty years."

Dr. Gary Goldman has been concerned about the risk associated with shingles, a disease that usually shows up in persons over fifty years of age. He has found a high incidence of shingles in children following widespread use of the varicella vaccine. Goldman has questioned whether it is more beneficial for chicken pox to remain active in the community so that adults could get a boostering effect from children with chicken pox. This could actually help to suppress the incidence of shingles in adulthood. This lack of natural boostering through children with chicken pox precipitated a possible need for a shingles vaccine—the VZV vaccine. This vaccine reduced the incidence of shingles by 50 percent. However, as the use of the varicella vaccine has increased, shingles incidence among adults increased 90 percent from 1998 to 2003. Goldman states in his published commentary, "The Case Against Universal Varicella Vaccination," "The 50 deaths (out of 4 million) per year that Varicella causes in children is quite low. In perspective, a person has a greater chance of dying by being struck by lightning in the United States (mean of 90 cases annually in the United States) than of a child's dying from contracting Varicella."

SERIOUS REACTIONS: WHAT TO LOOK FOR, WHAT TO DO

According to the CDC, moderate or severe reactions to a varicella vaccine should be reported to and checked by a doctor immediately. If any of these reactions were to occur, they would happen within a few minutes to a few hours after the shot. High fever and seizures could happen one to six weeks after the shot. All adverse reactions should also be reported to the Vaccine Adverse Events Reporting System (VAERS), which is explained in chapter 22. Signs to look for include:

- High fever
- Seizures
- Difficulty breathing
- Hoarseness or wheezing
- Weakness
- Fast heartbeat
- Dizziness
- Hives
- Paleness

BOTTOM LINE

Barbara Loe Fisher, co-founder and president of the National Vaccine Information Center, stated in 2000, "The Varicella vaccine should not be mandated," yet many states do require it for admission to school. After weighing the facts and looking at your options, only you can decide if you want your child to get the chicken pox vaccine.

In my practice, I do not recommend giving this vaccine as a routine to toddlers. This can present a problem since few children now get chicken pox because so many are vaccinated. If your child reaches twelve years of age and has not had the disease, it might be a good idea to have the child tested to see if there is immunity. The child could have had chicken pox that was not really evident and may be immune for life. If the titer is negative, indicating no immunity, consider giving the vaccine so that he or she will not have the disease at a later age—which may be more serious than having it as a young child.

Before you take your child in for his or her chicken pox shot, carefully review the list of "Who Should Not Get the Varicella Vaccine" in this chapter. Also, follow the suggestions listed at the end of chapter 21 to help protect your child against possible reactions to the vaccine. Varicella is not a benign vaccine.

NOTES

Centers for Disease Control and Prevention. Vaccine Information Statements. May 4, 2000.

FDA Consumer, September 1995. At www.fda.gov/fdac/features/795 chickpox.html.

Fisher, Barbara Loe. *The Consumer's Guide to Childhood Vaccines.* Vienna, VA: National Vaccine Information Center, 1997.

Press release from Barbara Loe Fisher, September 13, 2000.

Goldman, G. "The Case Against Universal Varicella Vaccination." *International Journal of Toxicology* 25 (2006): 313–17.

———. *The Chicken Pox Vaccine: A New Epidemic of Disease and Corruption.* Virtualbookworm.com (2006).

National Vaccine Information Center. *The Vaccine Reaction* (May 1995).

Needle Tips, October 2007. Immunization Action Coalition: www.immunize.org.

Plotkin, Stanley, et al. "Zoster in Normal Children After Varicella Vaccine." *Journal of Infectious Diseases* 159, no. 5 (May 1989): 1000–1001.

Wirrell, E., et al. "Stroke After Varicella Vaccination." *Journal of Pediatrics* 145, no. 6 (2004): 845–47.

www.cdc.gov/vaccines/pubs/ACIP-list.htm.

Chapter 12

❁

Hepatitis A

Hepatitis A, like its cousins hepatitis B and C, is a disease that causes inflammation of the liver. It is caused by the hepatitis A virus (HAV). Each year, an estimated 180,000 people in the United States get hepatitis A, yet about half of them don't even know they have it because they don't experience symptoms. About one hundred people die of liver disease caused by hepatitis A every year. Hepatitis A does not cause chronic infection and rarely causes death.

Hepatitis A is most common among children, which is not surprising, given the way it is spread—in the stool. It is difficult to keep children's hands clean, especially in social settings like day care where they interact and share toys. The virus can also spread through contaminated water and when someone with dirty hands prepares food. On rare occasions, it is transferred through donated blood.

Like chicken pox, hepatitis A is a much more serious disease in adults than it is in children. Seventy percent of adolescents and adults with hepatitis A get symptoms compared with only 30 percent of preschool-aged children.

Who Is at Risk for Hepatitis A?

Hepatitis A affects children much more than it does adults. Children, however, are less symptomatic than older adults. People most at risk for contracting hepatitis A include:

- Those who live in regions or communities largely populated by Native Americans, including Alaska, Hawaii, and the Pacific islands.
- People who live in eleven Western states, where half of all reported cases occur: Arizona, Alaska, Oregon, New Mexico, Utah, Idaho, Washington, Oklahoma, South Dakota, Nevada, and California.
- Anyone two years of age and older who is traveling or working in countries that have high hepatitis A rates, including those in Central and South America, Mexico, Asia (except Japan), Africa, and Southern or Eastern Europe.
- Those who use street drugs.
- Those who have chronic liver disease.
- Men who engage in homosexual activities.
- People who receive clotting factor concentrates.

Symptoms and Treatment

Once the HAV enters the body, it reproduces for about one month before liver damage becomes evident. The symptoms include jaundice, loss of appetite, dark urine, fever, and nausea. These symptoms last for up to two months for most people, but up to 15 percent of people will experience them on and off for about six months.

Hepatitis A Vaccine

The hepatitis A vaccine contains whole viruses killed by formaldehyde. The vaccine is licensed for use only in people who are two years of age or older and should not be taken by anyone who has had a serious allergic reaction to a previous dose of the vaccine. The vaccine's impact on pregnant women is not known, although the CDC believes the risk is very low. The CDC also says that anyone who has a moderate or severe illness should wait until they recover to get the vaccine but that mild illness is not a reason to wait. I routinely advise that people who have any level of illness should wait until they are better before getting the vaccine.

The CDC recommends that two doses of the vaccine be given at least six months apart to all one-year-old children. There is also a recommendation for vaccination of all children and adolescents age two years and older who live in a state, county, or community with a routine vaccination program already in place. In addition, the recommendation covers children traveling anywhere except the United States, Western Europe, New Zealand, Australia, Canada, and Japan; those who wish to be protected from hepatitis A infection; those who have chronic liver disease or clotting factor disorders; and male adolescents engaging in gay sex.

Adverse Reactions to the Vaccine

The CDC reports the vaccine is associated with a few negative reactions. They typically occur three to five days after vaccination and last for one or two days. They include:

- Soreness at the injection sight: affects 1 out of 2 adults, and up to 1 out of 5 children.
- Headache: 1 out of 6 adults and 1 out of 20 children.
- Loss of appetite: about 1 out of 12 children.

Serious allergic reactions, which the CDC says are very rare, may occur within a few minutes to a few hours of receiving the vaccination. Symptoms include wheezing, hives, paleness, weakness, a fast heartbeat, dizziness, and difficulty breathing. The vaccine manufacturer in its product insert also lists more severe reported adverse events such as convulsions, neuropathy, Guillain-Barré syndrome, multiple sclerosis, and other immune and brain complications. If these symptoms occur, a doctor should be contacted immediately, and the event should be reported to the Vaccine Adverse Events Reporting System.

An Alternative to the Vaccine

For people who do not live where possible exposure to HAV is constant but who have been exposed to the virus or may be exposed because of travel into an infected area, there is an alternative to the vaccine. Immune globulin provides protection for three to five months, depending on the dosage. Immune globulin, a type of antibody, should be given before or within two weeks of exposure to HAV. Side effects or risks associated with immune globulin are rare and may include swelling at the injection site, hives, or allergic reactions.

BOTTOM LINE

In my practice, I do not recommend hepatitis A vaccine as a routine inoculation for all children. It may be a consideration for those at higher risk (per CDC recommendation, above) or for those living in an endemic area for the disease. This is another vaccine grown in human fetal tissue, which could open the door for more reactions. It also contains formalin, phenoxyethanol, and albumin.

There are no adequate long-term studies for safety in vaccine recipients. The Merck package insert mentions a five-day period for fever and local complaints.

Notes

Immunization Action Coalition Web site: www.immunize.org.
Physicians' Desk Reference, 2008 vaccine package inserts.
Plotkin, S., P. Offit, and W. Orenstein. *Vaccines.* Philadelphia: Saunders, 2008.
www.cdc.gov/vaccines/pubs/ACIP-list.htm.

Chapter 13

❖

Pneumococcal Disease

THE BACTERIA THAT CAUSE PNEUMOCOCCAL DISEASE, *Strep-tococcus pneumoniae,* are a family of organisms that many people recognize by the abbreviated name *strep*. But don't let the short name fool you: This family has at least ninety different strains of the bacterium pneumococcus. Pneumococcus is responsible for a wide range of medical problems every year in the United States, including:

- Up to 570,000 cases of bacterial pneumonia (about 20 percent occur in infants and young children).
- Sixty-one thousand cases of bacteremia (bacteria in the bloodstream that can cause pneumonia, high fever, or meningitis). About sixteen thousand cases occur in children under age five.
- Seven million cases of ear infections in infants and young children.
- Up to three thousand cases of meningitis, of which about fourteen hundred cases occur in children younger than age

five. Up to 50 percent of children with meningitis suffer brain damage or hearing loss, and about 10 percent die.

What Is Pneumococcal Disease?

Of the more than ninety strains of pneumococcus bacteria, ten are believed to cause more than 60 percent of diseases around the world. Not all strains are found everywhere, and not all of them affect the same age groups. For example, currently there are seven strains (many antibiotic-resistant) responsible for about 80 percent of the pneumococcal infections in the United States in children younger than six years old.

Pneumococci live in the throat and nose of many people who don't become ill from the bacteria. These folks spread the disease when they sneeze, cough, or speak, and the droplets that get into the air are inhaled by a susceptible person. The bacteria then enter the bloodstream, which carries them to the brain or lungs.

Who Is at Risk for Pneumococcal Disease?

The majority of people who get pneumococcal disease are children younger than two years of age: 145 cases per 100,000 children aged two and younger. The next group at risk are adults older than seventy-four (54 cases per 100,000). The rate for all ages in between is 5 to 25 per 100,000.

Also at risk are adults who have any of the following conditions:

- Alcoholism
- Diabetes
- Kidney or liver disease

- HIV or cancer
- Damaged spleen
- Airway damage due to air pollution or smoking
- Impaired gag reflex due to alcohol, drugs, or age

Adults who are undergoing chemotherapy or who are taking high doses of prednisone are also at risk of pneumococcal disease.

Pneumococcal disease is responsible for 30 to 60 percent or more of all middle-ear infections, a condition that affects 91 percent of children before they reach two years of age. It causes 13 to 19 percent of all bacterial meningitis cases and is the most common cause of the disease among children younger than five years. About 20 percent of people who get pneumococcal meningitis die, and 25 to 30 percent of those who survive have permanent disabilities, such as hearing loss, seizure disorders, or mental retardation.

Pneumococcal Vaccines

On February 17, 2000, a second vaccine to help prevent pneumococcal disease in children was approved by the FDA. This new seven-valent vaccine, Prevnar, joined Pneumovax, a twenty-three-polyvalent vaccine (produced from cultures from twenty-three strains of pneumococcus) that has been available since 1983, and is generally recommended for adults.

Prevnar is a conjugate vaccine (see chapter 1) and is effective in infants and children younger than two years. This vaccine is effective against the seven pneumococcal strains most responsible for the disease in infants and young children. However, it is not effective against eighty-three other pneumococcal strains. The FDA announced that the new vaccine prevents blood poisoning (bacteremia) and meningitis, but not ear infections. However, researchers did document a slight reduction in the number of ear infections during testing of the vaccine.

In 2007, some disturbing news emerged about the Prevnar vaccine. CDC researchers found an increase in the rates of pneumococcal infections not covered by the current pneumococcal vaccine among children in Alaska. There are at least two other pneumococcal vaccines in study for use in children, one containing nine of the ninety types of pneumococcal bacteria and one containing eleven.

RECOMMENDED DOSING SCHEDULES

The CDC's Advisory Committee on Immunization Practices (ACIP) recommends that all children younger than age two receive the Prevnar pneumococcal vaccine. The vaccine is given in a series of four shots at two months, four months, six months, and between twelve and fifteen months. For babies and children who start the series later, the number of shots is reduced because the manufacturer found that a child's response improves with age, so children who start the series later need fewer shots.

- Start between seven and eleven months: get three shots.
- One to two years: two shots.
- Two years: one shot.

The ACIP recommends that Prevnar also be given to children aged two to five if they are at high risk for pneumococcal disease. Native American and black children, as well as those with certain chronic illnesses, are considered to be at high risk.

Safety and Effectiveness

To test the safety and effectiveness of Prevnar, the manufacturer sponsored studies of thirty-eight thousand children in which the experimental pneumococcal vaccine was compared with an experimental meningococcal vaccine for safety and efficacy. Half the children received Prevnar along with Hib and DTP shots; the other half received Hib and DTP with meningococcal vaccine. The FDA reports that the Prevnar vaccine was 90 percent effective in preventing blood poisoning and pneumococcal meningitis.

Between 12 and 20 percent of children experienced tenderness, swelling, or redness at the injection site. Irritability, seizures, drowsiness, restless sleep, and fever were also more common in the Prevnar group. About one-third of the children had a temperature greater than one hundred degrees.

Although the FDA did not evaluate Prevnar for the prevention of pneumococcal ear infections, the number of chronic ear infections (defined as five or more episodes within six months or six or more episodes in twelve months) declined nearly 6 percent in the thirty-eight thousand children who participated in the trials.

Pneumovax, used primarily for adults, is effective against twenty-three types of pneumococcus, which are responsible for at least 90 percent of all pneumococcal disease seen in the United States. This vaccine is 56 to 81 percent effective in preventing pneumococcal disease and may be less effective in people who have a weakened immune system.

Published Study Using a Nine-Valent Pneumococcal Vaccine

The Gambia Pneumococcal Vaccine Trial studied the effects of using a nine-valent vaccine in children in a developing country. It was the first controlled vaccine clinical trial in twenty years to show a statistically significant reduction in overall child mortality. There was a 15 percent drop in hospitalizations after the vaccination, and in general there was reduced death and illness in the rural areas. This was published in the *Lancet* in 2005.

BOTTOM LINE

In my practice, I do not recommend the use of the Prevnar vaccine for all children. There is some concern that we may be setting the stage for new super-bacteria that cause ear infections. Since the Prevnar only protects against seven of the ninety possible strains, the possibility exists for some of the eighty-three remaining strains to become resistant to antibiotics. This actually has already been seen in medical practice.

What I have used in my practice is the adult form of the pneumococcal vaccine, Pneumovax, which contains no thimerosal. This is effective against twenty-three of the ninety strains of the organism. I give a dose to children at two years of age and evaluate them for a booster in five to seven years. If a nine-valent or an eleven-valent vaccine is introduced, this would be a possibility for better coverage at an earlier age than two. Both are presently in study.

NOTES

Centers for Disease Control and Prevention. "Preventing Pneumococcal Disease Among Infants and Young Children." *Morbidity and Mortality Weekly Report* 49, no. RR-9 (October 6, 1999): 1–35.

Cutts, F. T. "Efficacy of the Nine-Valent Pneumococcal Conjugate Vaccine Against Pneumonia and Invasive Pneumococcal Disease in the Gambia Randomized, Double Blind Placebo Controlled Trial." *Lancet* 365, no. 946J (2005): 1139–46.

Fisher, Barbara Loe. *The Consumer's Guide to Childhood Vaccines.* Vienna, VA: National Vaccine Information Center, 1997.

Humiston, S., and C. Good. *Vaccinating Your Child: Questions and Answers for the Concerned Parent.* Atlanta: Peachtree Publishers, 2000, 135–71.

National Vaccine Information Center Web site: www.nvic.org.

"The New Meningitis/Pneumococcal Vaccine Called PREVNAR." www.thekcrachannel.com/sh/health/stories/health-20000218-183809.html.

"Prevnar and Ear Infection Efficacy." www.babycenter.com/topic 11290.html.

www.cdc.gov/vaccines/recs/provisional/default.htm#acip.

Chapter 14

❁

Meningococcal Disease

Meningococcal disease, like pneumococcal disease, can cause meningitis in people of all ages. This often deadly disease can be prevented with a vaccine. Unlike pneumococcal disease, however, meningococcal disease is caused by a different organism, and does not affect nearly as many individuals: Between twenty-four hundred and three thousand people in the United States get meningococcal disease each year. That's about 1 in every 100,000 people, compared with 23 per 100,000 for pneumococcal disease.

Between 10 and 13 percent of those in the United States who contract meningococcal disease die each year, even if they receive antibiotics early in the course of the disease. Among those who survive, 3 to 15 percent experience severe complications, including mental retardation, loss of limbs, renal problems, and hearing loss.

What Is Meningococcal Disease?

Meningococcal disease is caused by *Neisseria meningitidis,* an organism that causes meningitis (an infection of the brain's outer lining) and meningococcemia (blood infection, or blood poisoning). Like pneumococcal disease, meningococcal disease is spread in air droplets that are released from the nose or throat of infected people when they sneeze, cough, or talk. Between 5 and 11 percent of adults have meningococcus in the lining of their nose or throat.

Who Is at Risk for Meningococcal Disease?

In October 1999, the Advisory Committee on Immunization Practices (ACIP) modified its guidelines for the use of the meningococcal vaccine, and recommended it be given especially to college freshmen who live in dormitories. This group is at increased risk for meningococcal disease compared with other people their age.

The ACIP based its recommendation on two studies done by the CDC in 1998, which found a six- to sevenfold higher risk for the disease among college freshmen compared with all college students. Although anyone can become infected with *Neisseria meningitidis,* research shows that excessive alcohol consumption, exposure to active and passive smoking, and patronizing bars appear to increase students' risk for the disease. Even among college students, however, meningococcal disease is very rare. The vaccine is now recommended for children aged eleven and older.

RECOMMENDED DOSING

The recent CDC guidelines for dosing are as follows:

Give one dose of the meningococcal vaccine (MCV4) to adolescents aged eleven through eighteen years.

Vaccinate all college freshmen living in dorms who have not been vaccinated.

Vaccinate all children aged two years and older who have any of the following risk factors (use the polysaccharide vaccine MPSV if age younger than eleven, or conjugate MCV4 for those eleven and older):

- Anatomic or functional asplenia (without a spleen).
- Terminal complement component deficiencies (immune problems).
- Travel to or residence in countries in which meningococcal disease is hyperendemic or epidemic (such as sub-Saharan Africa).

How Effective Is the Vaccine?

The vaccine currently available protects against only some of the types (called serogroups) of the meningococcus bacterium, and none of them completely. Thirteen meningococcal organism subgroups and five serotypes (A, B, C, Y, and W-135) are responsible for nearly all cases of the disease worldwide. In the United States serotypes B, C, and Y cause the majority of the cases. The vaccination significantly reduces the risk of meningococcal disease caused by the serogroups A, C, Y, and W-135, but it does not protect against serogroup B, which causes about 30 percent of all cases of the disease in all age categories. Menactra, one of the available vaccines, was licensed in 2005, and the CDC recommends it for eleven- to eighteen-year-olds. It does not protect against type B, which causes a third of all cases in the US and more than half of cases in infants. Menactra actually offers zero protection against meningococcal disease a third to half the time depending on the age of the person. It is only effective for three to five years.

Disease Outbreaks: 1980 to 1996

Between 1980 and 1993, there were twenty-one outbreaks of meningococcal disease, three of which occurred on college campuses. From 1994 to 1996, an additional twenty-six outbreaks occurred, four in colleges. Researchers note that the majority of cases among college students are caused by either serotype C, Y, or W-135, which are all preventable with the vaccine. The latest available data show that serogroups C and Y caused about 70 percent of cases of meningococcal disease among college students in 1998–99.

RISKS ASSOCIATED WITH MENINGOCOCCAL VACCINES

- Guillain-Barré syndrome.
- Various side effects when given with the human papilloma virus (HPV) vaccine (according to current CDC recommendation):

  1. Guillain-Barré syndrome increased by 1000 percent.
  2. Respiratory problems increased by 114 percent.
  3. Cardiac problems increased by 118 percent.
  4. Neuromuscular problems increased by 234 percent.
  5. Convulsions and neurological problems increased by 301 percent.

The Vaccine Adverse Effects Reporting System's records through November 2008 showed 1,667 emergency room visits and six deaths related to the Menactra vaccine.

BOTTOM LINE

In my practice, I do not recommend giving the Menactra vaccine to children until they go to college unless they are in a boarding school or a group home. If there have been any reported cases of meningococcal disease in the community, I usually recommend one dose for eleven- to eighteen-year-olds of a non-thimerosal-containing vaccine. At the time of this writing, there is some new information about an increased risk of Guillain-Barré syndrome with the use of the Menactra vaccine. As with any emerging information, parents need to weigh the possible side effects against the benefits of the vaccine before agreeing to let it be given to their child or adolescent.

NOTES

American Academy of Family Physicians, editorial by James C. Turner, M.D. "Meningococcal Vaccine for College Freshmen." August 1, 2000. www.aafp.org/afp/200000801/editorials.html.

Erickson, L., and P. De Wals. "Complications and Sequelae of Meningococcal Disease in Quebec, Canada, 1990–1994." *Clinical Infectious Diseases* 26 (1998): 1159–64.

http://articles.mercola.com/sites/articles/archive/2007/10/06/doctors-in-denial-about-vaccine-reactions.aspx.

Immunization Action Coalition Advisory Committee on Immunization Practices Web site: www.immunize.org/acip.

National Vaccine Information Center Med Alerts (Vaccine Adverse Event Reporting System—VAERS—information up through January 2009).

National Vaccine Information Center Web site: www.nvic.org.

www.cdc.gov/epo/mmwr/preview/mmwrhtml/rr4907a2.htm.

www.cdc.gov/vaccines/pubs/ACIP-listl.htm.

Chapter 15

❀

Influenza

EVERY FALL, THE CALL GOES OUT FROM FEDERAL HEALTH agency officials: *Get your flu shot.* While the flu is merely a nuisance or minor inconvenience to many people, for some, including the elderly and anyone with a weakened immune system, it can cause serious complications, even death.

In fact, flu epidemics over the centuries have killed millions of people. One of the deadliest occurred in 1918 and 1919: Twenty million people died around the world, half a million in the United States alone. Officials got a scare in 1997 when a flu strain that had previously affected only birds, mostly chickens, killed a child in Hong Kong. Scientists scrambled to develop a vaccine. The Hong Kong government then ordered that 1.5 million chickens be destroyed to prevent the flu strain from spreading. These drastic measures apparently worked, as that particular viral strain did not return. But different strains of the flu return each year, affecting millions of people around the world. Most people do not die of the flu, but many do end up in the hospital.

Influenza is a group of viruses that can cause several different complications, including pneumonia and myocarditis (inflammation of the heart). Symptoms usually come on quickly and include headache, runny or stuffy nose, chills, dry cough, sore throat, fever, muscle aches, and exhaustion. Very young children who get the flu sometimes experience nausea and vomiting, but these symptoms are rare in adults. Flu symptoms typically last for several days, but among the elderly they can linger for weeks.

Flu viruses live in the nose, throat, and lungs of infected individuals, who spread these germs in the form of droplets in the air when they talk, sneeze, or cough. Susceptible people inhale these droplets or pick them up from objects that infected people have handled. These viruses result in hospitalization for about 110,000 people in the United States each year.

Who Is at Risk for the Flu?

Children aged five to fourteen have the highest infection rate for flu, but the elderly have the highest rate of flu-related deaths: 90 percent of flu deaths occur in this population. Elderly people who reside in long-term care facilities are at particular risk. Beginning in 2000, the CDC lowered the beginning age at which older people should get the vaccine from sixty-five years to fifty.

Other people at risk for the flu include those who have diabetes, heart disease, lung disease, asthma, anemia and other blood disorders, kidney dysfunction, or those who have a compromised immune system.

The Flu Vaccine

Flu vaccines are prepared from the fluids of chick embryos that are inoculated (injected) with specific types of influenza virus. Manufacturers then add formaldehyde to inactivate the viruses and thimerosal to preserve the vaccine.

Creating flu vaccines is an educated guessing game. Every year, a group of federal health officials get together and try to guess which three strains of influenza are most likely to cause the most problems in the following year.

FEDERAL/STATE GUIDELINES FOR INFLUENZA DOSING

The CDC recommends that the trivalent inactivated flu vaccine (TIV) be given to the following individuals:

- Persons six months or older, including school-aged children, wanting to reduce their risk of becoming ill with flu or of spreading it to others.
- All children aged six through eighteen years (this is a new recommendation as of 2008) as well as siblings and household contacts of these children.
- Persons aged five years and older who have a risk factor. These include pregnancy, heart disease, lung disease, diabetes, renal dysfunction, hemoglobinopathy, immunosupression, and long-term aspirin therapy. Also at risk are those with a condition that compromises respiratory function, requires the handling of respiratory secretions, or can increase the risk of aspiration.
- Those who live in a chronic care facility.

- Persons who live or work with at-risk people as listed above.

The CDC recommends the live attenuated influenza vaccine (LAIV) nasal spray for healthy, nonpregnant persons aged five through forty-nine years. Those aged six months through eight years who are receiving the vaccine for the first time can receive two doses of either TIV (four weeks apart) or LAIV (six weeks apart)

The flu vaccine should not be given within three days of the DTaP.

Who Should Not Get the Vaccine?

Persons with previous anaphylaxis to this vaccine, to any of its components, or to eggs should not receive the vaccine.

The live attenuated influenza vaccine should not be given to those with the following conditions:

- Pregnancy
- Asthma, reactive airways disease, or other chronic disorder of the pulmonary or cardiovascular system
- An underlying medical condition, including metabolic diseases such as diabetes, renal dysfunction, and hemoglobinopathy
- Known or suspected immune deficiency disease or current immunosuppressive therapy
- A history of Guillain-Barré syndrome

Those people suffering moderate or severe illness, and those with a history of Guillain-Barré syndrome, should not get the trivalent inactivated flu vaccine within six weeks of receiving a prior dose of TIV.

How Effective Are Flu Vaccines?

The effectiveness of flu vaccines changes from year to year. If health officials accurately anticipate the specific flu strains likely to be problematic, the vaccine can be 70 to 80 percent effective in temporarily preventing flu in people who are younger than sixty-five years of age. For people older than sixty-five, efficacy is only 30 to 40 percent in preventing the flu—but the vaccine is believed to be 50 to 60 percent effective in preventing pneumonia and hospitalization and 80 percent effective in preventing death from flu. If the officials do not guesstimate well, effectiveness can be even lower for all categories. Dr. Tom Jefferson's study in the *British Medical Journal* in 2006 showed the flu shot to be only mildly effective in the elderly. In 2005, a study published in the *Archives of Internal Medicine* suggested that influenza-related mortality decline in the 1970s among people aged sixty-five through seventy-four came from immunity acquired during the pandemic of 1968. Another study in the *Lancet,* 2008, examined 1,173 elderly people with community-acquired pneumonia and 2,346 controls. The study found no link between the flu vaccine and reduced risk of illness.

Some people have the misconception that getting a flu shot will prevent them from getting various gastrointestinal, ear, and respiratory infections. Flu vaccines focus on three influenza viruses only and offer no protection against other infections. Because it takes about two weeks after receiving a flu vaccine for it to work, you can get the flu if you were already infected at the time you got the vaccine.

Public officials are still trying to justify the distribution of the influenza vaccine to the masses; the CDC is running several studies toward this end. What seems to be understood is that the flu vaccine is less effective in the elderly and in very young children. In the 2008–9 season, more than 143 million doses of the vaccine were administered.

The CDC recommendation that healthy children should get

a flu vaccine raises questions for many people. Mass vaccination of healthy children removes natural antibodies to the flu, which are provided when the flu is acquired naturally. Medical science is not yet certain whether it is better for healthy children, who rarely experience complications from flu, to get the flu and develop natural, permanent immunity to that specific flu strain, or for them to get vaccinated every year and suppress flu. The state of California saw a decline in cases of autism after thimerosal was reduced in most vaccines. Following the recommendation to give the flu shot to children and pregnant women, however, the numbers again began to rise. Dr. Tom Jefferson published a study in the *British Medical Journal* in 2009 that questioned the quality of studies regarding vaccines appearing in prestigious journals. It was stated in the article that "influenza vaccination continues to be recommended globally, despite growing doubts about the validity of the scientific evidence underpinning policy recommendations."

Adverse Reactions

The CDC reports that the most common reactions are mild and usually begin within twelve hours of receiving the flu vaccination. They include fever, aches, and soreness, swelling, or redness at the injection site and usually last one to two days. Because the viruses used in the vaccine are killed, they cannot cause influenza.

More severe problems such as life-threatening allergic reactions are very rare, reports the CDC. However, if symptoms do occur (difficulty breathing, rash, fast heartbeat, dizziness, weakness, paleness, or wheezing), they usually appear within a few minutes to a few hours after the shot. A doctor should be contacted immediately, and the adverse reactions should be reported to the Vaccine Adverse Events Reporting System.

Another serious reaction to the flu vaccine is Guillain-Barré syndrome (see chapter 5). Most people recover at least partially but have some permanent disability from the disease. Less than 5 percent of cases result in death. The CDC estimates that the risk of getting Guillain-Barré syndrome from a flu vaccine is 1 or 2 cases per 1 million people vaccinated.

BOTTOM LINE

In my practice, I do not recommend the influenza vaccine for children and pregnant women. The package insert states that it is "not known whether influenza virus vaccine can cause fetal harm when administered to a pregnant woman." It is amazing to me that with all the controversy about the dangers of thimerosal, some brands of flu vaccine are still sold with thimerosal as a preservative. Until thimerosal is removed from the flu vaccine, I have concerns about its safety. I believe the ethyl mercury in the vaccine can cause neurological or immune system problems for anyone who gets the shot, especially the elderly. Speak with your doctor about whether the vaccine's benefits outweigh the possible risks. There are some influenza vaccines available that are thimerosal-free.

NOTES

Elliott, V. "Research at Odds Over Impact of Flu Vaccine." *American Medical News* 52, no. 4 (January 26, 2009).

Immunization Action Coalition Advisory Committee on Immunization Practices: www.immunize.org/acip.

Jackson, L., et al. *Lancet* "Influenza Vaccination and Risk of a Community-Acquired Pneumonia in Immunocompetent Elderly People: A Population-Based, Nested, Case-Control Study." (August 2, 2008).

Jefferson, T. "Relation of Study Quality, Concordance, Take Home

Message, Findings, and Impact in Studies of Influenza Vaccines: Systematic Review." *British Medical Journal* (2009): 338–54.

———. *British Medical Journal* "Influenza Vaccination: Policy versus Evidence" (October 28, 2006).

Physicians' Desk Reference, package insert for vaccine, 2008.

www.cdc.gov/vaccines/pubs/ACIP-list.htm.

Chapter 16

❄

Rotavirus

Rᴏᴛᴀᴠɪʀᴜꜱ ɪꜱ ᴛʜᴇ ᴍᴏꜱᴛ ᴄᴏᴍᴍᴏɴ ᴄᴀᴜꜱᴇ ᴏꜰ ꜱᴇᴠᴇʀᴇ ɢᴀꜱᴛʀᴏ-enteritis in infants and young children. The disease may cause diarrhea, dehydration, vomiting, and fever. Almost all children have been infected by age five. Annually, in the United States, Rotavirus is responsible for 3 million infections, more than 400,000 physician visits, 160,000 emergency department visits, 55,000 to 70,000 hospitalizations, and between 20 and 60 deaths.

FEDERAL/STATE GUIDELINES FOR DOSING ROTAVIRUS VACCINE

The recommendation is to give a three-dose series at age two months, four months, and six months.

- Dose 1 may be given as early as six weeks of age.
- Dose 3 is to be given no later than age thirty-two weeks.

- The series is not to be started in infants older than twelve weeks.
- Doses 2 and 3 may be given four weeks after the previous dose.

Who Should Not Get the Vaccine?

- Those with previous anaphylaxis to the vaccine or to any of its components.
- Children with moderate or severe illness.
- Children with altered immunocompetence.
- Children with moderate to severe gastroenteritis or chronic gastrointestinal disease.
- Children with a history of intussusception.

Adverse Reactions

The Vaccine Adverse Events Reporting System received 1,901 reports of adverse events after RotaTeq vaccination between February 1, 2006, and September 25, 2007. One hundred sixty intussusception reports were confirmed. Forty-nine percent occurred in the first twenty-one days following the vaccination with RotaTeq; twenty-seven cases occurred within seven days. With the previous rotavirus vaccine, 60 percent occurred between one and seven days after the vaccination. The CDC has said that the observed rate of intussusceptions was not higher than the age-adjusted background rate of the condition. In other words, the CDC does not feel that the RotaTeq vaccine should be taken off the market because of these side effects.

BOTTOM LINE

In my practice, I do not recommend this vaccine as a routine part of the infant vaccine series. It is a live, viral vaccine. The rotavirus illness is not severe enough to warrant three doses of such a vaccine, and one of the major side effects of the vaccine is exactly what we are trying to stop—diarrhea.

NOTES

Immunization Action Coalition Advisory Committee on Immunization Practices Web site (2009 archive): www.immunize.org/acip_asp.2009.

Waknine, Yael. Medscape, February 14, 2007.

www.cdc.gov/vaccines/pubs/ACIP-list.htm, 2009.

www.cdc.gov/vaccinesafety/vaers/rotateq.htm, 2009.

Chapter 17

❁

Human Papilloma Virus

Human papilloma virus (HPV) can cause genital warts and cervical cancer. There are many types of HPV virus, more than fifteen of which can cause cervical cancer. It is important to note that the human papilloma virus is not only transmitted sexually. There have been cases documented in children and women who have never been sexually active.

HPV is the most commonly sexually transmitted infection in the United States. More than twenty million men and women in the US are infected. It is most common in the late teens and early twenties. By age fifty, at least 80 percent of sexually active women will have acquired HPV. The virus is responsible for nearly 100 percent of cervical cancers in women. Cervical cancer is diagnosed in more than ninety-seven hundred women in the US yearly and results in thirty-seven hundred deaths.

The Human Papilloma Virus Vaccine

Gardasil, Merck's HPV vaccine, protects against four strains of HPV, two of which cause genital warts, numbers 6 and 11. The other two, HPV 16 and 18, are cancer-causing viruses. These cause 70 percent of cervical cancers. The vaccine was approved in 2006 by the FDA and was recommended in June 2006 for females aged nine to twenty-six by the Centers for Disease Control's Advisory Committee on Immunization Practices (ACIP).

This is not a cancer cure but a disease preventive. It really has not been proven to prevent cancer—studies have not run long enough to determine that. It may take fifteen years to develop a cancer. The vaccine would have to be in use at least that long to prove whether or not it prevents cancer. It will not protect someone who has already contracted the virus.

In a May 18, 2006, Background Document for the FDA Vaccines and Related Biological Products Advisory Committee (VRBPAC), the FDA staff stated that the Merck clinical trial data indicated that there may be "the potential for Gardasil to enhance cervical disease in subjects who had evidence of persistent infection with vaccine-related HPV types prior to the vaccination." This could mean that a young woman with HPV disease before getting the vaccine may actually be more at risk for cervical cancer if she is given the vaccine. Only time will tell. It might be noted that females who are now being vaccinated with Gardasil are not routinely being tested for active HPV infection before vaccination. To test for HPV, one would have to do a vaginal swab, which is difficult and inappropriate for young girls.

One of the critics of the way that the vaccine has been marketed is Diane M. Harper, who is a scientist, physician, professor, and the director of the Gynecologic Cancer Prevention Research Group at the Norris Cotton Cancer Center at Dartmouth Medical School in New Hampshire. Dr. Harper has spent twenty years developing the vaccine for the human papilloma virus.

Dr. Harper stated in an interview that the vaccine is not for young girls and that it has not been tested for effectiveness in them. Administering it to young girls may not protect them; in the worst-case scenario, instead of serving to reduce the numbers of cervical cancers within twenty-five years, such a vaccination crusade could actually cause the numbers to go up.

Gardasil and the State Legislatures

Female legislators began introducing legislation in a number of states that would mandate the vaccine for eleven- to twelve-year-old girls. More than twenty-five states are considering some form of legislation requiring the new vaccine for young girls. In February 2006, Governor Rick Perry of Texas personally mandated the Gardasil vaccine for eleven- to twelve-year-old girls in his state. This move met with fury in the parental ranks. The mandate failed.

So where does money play a part in this frenzy? The three-shot series costs $360. Merck sold $723 million worth of the Gardasil vaccine in the first half of 2007. In the same six months, Merck posted nearly $2 billion in revenue from vaccines alone. But should big business profit be the driving factor in marketing a vaccine that could have a positive effect on cervical cancer prevention but instead may have a devastating effect on the health of young girls?

FEDERAL/STATE GUIDELINES FOR DOSING THE HUMAN PAPILLOMA VIRUS VACCINE

The recommendation is to give a three-dose series to girls at age eleven to twelve years on a zero-, two-, six-

month schedule. (It may be given as young as nine years
of age.)

All older girls and women through twenty-six years
who were not vaccinated previously should be vaccinated.

- Dose 2 may by given four weeks after dose 1.
- Dose 3 may be given twelve weeks after dose 2.

Who Should Not Get the Vaccine?

- Pregnant women.
- Women who test positive for HPV prior to the vaccination.
- Women suffering moderate or severe acute illness.
- Those with previous anaphylaxis to this vaccine or to any of
  its components.

Reported Side Effects

By May 11, 2007, 1,637 adverse vaccination reactions were
reported to the FDA related to Gardasil via the Vaccine Adverse
Event Reporting System (VAERS). These included 371 serious reactions. Forty-two pregnant women received the vaccine.
Eighteen had side effects ranging from spontaneous abortion to
fetal abnormalities.

Other reported side effects include fainting, dizziness, nausea, pain, itching, paralysis, Bell's palsey, Guillain-Barré syndrome, and seizures. VAERS reports through November 2008
for Gardasil-related reactions included 5,021 emergency room
visits, 2,017 who did not recover from symptoms, 9 cardiac ar-
rests, 23 blood clots, 544 seizures, 16 strokes, and 29 deaths.

BOTTOM LINE

In my practice, I do not recommend this vaccine—especially for young girls between the ages of nine and eighteen years of age. There clearly has not been enough safety study. One of my concerns is that the women who take the vaccine may not continue to do Pap smears as a true preventive measure for cervical cancer. This vaccine does not take the place of the Pap smear, and it is not beneficial at least a third of the time because it does not cover all of the types of HPV that can cause cancer.

There are too many unanswered questions about this vaccine. The side effect profile is significant and the question of whether it really prevents cervical cancer has not been answered. The risk is too great when we already have a very effective tool to detect cervical changes before cancer develops—the Pap smear. I believe that we can still depend on it as the best preventive measure against cervical cancer.

NOTES

Bevington, Cindy. "Researcher Blasts HPV Marketing." www.laleva. org, March 14, 2007.

Centers for Disease Control. Reports of Health Concerns Following HPV Vaccination, October 21, 2008. www.cdc.gov/vaccinesafety/ vaers/gardasil.htm.

News release by NVIC, February 21, 2007. National Vaccine Information Center: www.nvic.org.

Vaccine Adverse Event Reporting System (VAERS), May 2007. www. medalerts.org.

Chapter 18

❈

Vaccines for World Travelers

Some foreign countries require that you have certain vaccinations before you enter or leave. Because each country has different requirements and the necessary vaccines may need to be taken in a series spanning weeks or months, gather information about vaccine requirements several months before your departure. That includes being up to date on routine shots, such as measles, mumps, rubella, hepatitis B, and chicken pox. You may also need to get hepatitis A, flu, meningococcus, and rabies vaccines, depending on your destination.

Here is a brief review of some of the common vaccines you may need if you are traveling overseas. Please consult your state or local health department for more details on vaccines for travelers—especially for infants and young children.

JAPANESE ENCEPHALITIS

Japanese encephalitis is a viral disease characterized by inflammation of the brain. It is spread by a bite from the culex mosquito, which lives in parts of rural, agricultural Asia and India. The disease is rare in Americans: Between 1978 and 1992, only eleven cases were reported among US citizens living or traveling in Asia. Fewer than one in one million unvaccinated Americans who visited Asia have gotten the disease.

Symptoms of the disease include headache, fever, lethargy, vomiting, diarrhea, seizure, and coma. Only 1 out of 250 infected people have symptoms, and 5 to 30 percent of people die. Between 30 and 50 percent of survivors have permanent damage, including convulsions, memory loss, paralysis, or behavioral problems.

People who should consider getting the vaccine are those who will be spending a month or longer in high-risk areas of Asia, India, or the western Pacific. The vaccine is given in three doses over a five-week period. It is about 80 percent effective.

Adverse reactions include pain, swelling, and redness at the injection site in about 20 percent of people. About 10 percent experience malaise, headache, dizziness, vomiting, fever, rash, abdominal pain, or muscle aches. Severe reactions are rare.

CHOLERA

The bacterium *Vibrio cholerae* that causes this disease is common in Central and South America, Africa, and Asia. The disease is carried in contaminated water and in fish and shellfish that has not been cooked properly. Cholera is usually found in poor regions rather than in tourist areas, where the water is treated and food is more carefully prepared. The disease is relatively rare, affecting only 1 in 500,000 Western travelers.

Cholera is characterized by diarrhea and vomiting. Only 2 to 5 percent of people get a severe case of the disease. Because the bacteria are destroyed by stomach acid, most people do not get symptoms unless they have consumed a great deal of contaminated water or food or they are taking antacids, which reduce stomach acid. People at highest risk are those who are taking anti-ulcer medication, as well as infants, young children, and people with liver disease or compromised immune systems.

No foreign country currently officially requires cholera vaccine for entry. However, parts of some African nations do locally demand proof of vaccination. In other cases, cholera vaccination may be helpful for people who will be in high-risk countries and who are taking antacids; for people who may be living in regions of poor sanitation for a long time (such as relief workers); and anyone who may not have access to reliable medical care.

The cholera vaccine is administered in one shot. An oral form, which is more effective, is not available in the United States. The vaccine is protective in about only 50 percent of people who get it. Most people who get the injection experience swelling, redness, and pain at the site, and these resolve within a few days. Fever, headache, and malaise occur frequently, but severe reactions are rare.

YELLOW FEVER

The *Aedes aeypti* mosquito carries the yellow fever virus, which can infect people who live or travel in northern South America and sub-Saharan Africa. Most people who are infected with the virus don't have symptoms, but those who do experience headache, fever, pain in the lower spine, extreme sensitivity to light, loss of appetite, and vomiting within three to six days of being bitten.

Up to 15 percent of infected individuals develop severe symptoms, including jaundice (a liver disease that causes the skin and eyes to turn yellow), bloody vomit and stools, and coma. Most people who reach this stage die.

The vaccine is virtually 100 percent effective and offers protection for about ten years, after which a booster is needed. A small percentage of people experience pain and redness at the injection site, or fever, mild headache, or muscle aches. Severe autoimmune and neurological reactions are rare. Because the vaccine is cultured in chick embryos, people who are allergic to eggs should not take the vaccine.

Some countries in South America and Africa require proof of vaccination to enter or even pass through the country. Contact your state or local health department for the latest requirements.

BOTTOM LINE

The vaccines discussed in this chapter are not required by state law, but you may be in a situation in which you or your child may need them. They are not covered by the National Childhood Vaccine Injury Act or the Vaccine Injury Compensation Program. For information on these vaccines, contact your state or local health department, and you may also want to gather information from the following organizations:

- International Society of Travel Medicine, www.istm.org
- American Society of Tropical Medicine and Hygiene, www.astmh.org
- International Association for Medical Assistance to Travelers, 716-754-4883
- American Citizens Services, 202-647-5225

Chapter 19

❖

Vaccines of the Future:
Sooner than You Think?

IMAGINE DRIVING YOUR TWELVE-YEAR-OLD SON OR DAUGHTER down to the doctor's office for a shot to help prevent sexually transmitted diseases (STDs). Sound impossible? Guess again. The Centers for Disease Control (CDC) already has plans to give vaccines for STDs such as chlamydia, herpes simplex, and Neisseria gonorrhea. The human papilloma virus vaccine is on the market. Others vaccines such as HIV/AIDS (human immunodeficiency virus/acquired immunodeficiency syndrome), cancer, and dozens of other diseases are being studied. Many of the vaccines in the pipeline are being recommended for infants and children, usually at age eleven to twelve years.

Interest in vaccine development has been vitalized in recent years for several reasons. One is the emergence of diseases such as AIDS. Another is the fact that many disease-causing organisms are becoming resistant to medications like antibiotics faster than scientists can create new drugs. Yet another reason is that new technology, especially genetic engineering, has opened up a whole new world for researchers looking for ways to fight disease. Genetically engineered vaccines, or recombinant DNA vaccines, are the wave of the future.

Although there are currently more than two hundred different vaccines in some state of development, in this chapter we will look at only a few of the most controversial and perhaps most imminent. But not all of those vaccines, and even some of those given today, will be given by injection. Researchers are looking at other ways to give vaccines, including via nasal spray, skin patch, and in food, as edible vaccines. These options are also discussed below.

HIV/AIDS VACCINE

In February 1997, members of the CDC's Advisory Committee on Immunization Practices (ACIP) gathered to do what they are charged to do: make vaccine policy for the United States. During that meeting, ACIP member Neal Halsey, M.D., chairman of the American Academy of Pediatrics Committee on Infectious Diseases, raised the topic of an HIV vaccine. He told the members that "We really see age eleven to twelve as the target age for introduction of vaccines for prevention of sexually transmitted diseases," and said "it would be nice" if they could plan to have studies ready "when you move another step in the direction of actually having a candidate vaccine." So today's parents of infants, toddlers, or young children may soon be faced with the possibility of getting an HIV vaccine for their kids.

Helping the ACIP make those steps was President Bill Clinton. In 1997, he announced that the National Institutes of Health would establish a new AIDS vaccine research center. He also challenged both the drug industry and researchers to develop an AIDS vaccine and make it available within ten years. If that challenge is met, parents who today have preschoolers could be among the first to bring their preteen children in for the vaccine.

Rocky Road to an HIV/AIDS Vaccine

There appear to be many candidates in the running for an HIV/AIDS vaccine. Since the first human trial for an AIDS vaccine began in 1987, more than forty other trials for experimental HIV vaccines have been launched, many of them in the United States. It is still too early to know how many—if any—of these will make it to the marketplace. That's because the road is littered with hurdles.

For example, drugs and vaccines are typically tested on animals before they advance to trials with humans. Yet so far there are no suitable animal models for testing the effectiveness and safety of the vaccines. Many of the monkeys that had been given live HIV vaccines have died or developed AIDS symptoms. Researchers also do not fully understand the origins and progress of the disease, which makes it difficult to prevent. There is also the problem with mutation: The disease undergoes almost continual changes, which makes the vaccines of little use from the start.

Two experts in AIDS research, Dr. Dennis Burton of the Scripps Research Institute in La Jolla, California, and Dr. John Moore of the Aaron Diamond AIDS Research Center at Rockefeller University in New York, explain that even when researchers have found vaccines that attack and destroy strains of HIV, other, resistant strains hide from the vaccines and continue reproducing HIV in the body. These renegade strains give birth to new strains, which are unaffected by any previous vaccines.

One place researchers may find an answer to how to make an HIV vaccine is in a population that is exposed to the disease but does not get it. Drs. Burton and Moore note that many African prostitutes are "highly exposed, yet HIV-uninfected," which leads scientists to wonder if they have some sort of natural immunity that is not yet understood. If such a natural immunity can be identified, researchers could be on their way to a vaccine. And because the threat of HIV/AIDS is so great (HIV infects one new person every six seconds, which is 5.8 million people per year), the search for a vaccine goes on despite the difficulties.

One interesting development coming out of the HIV/AIDS vaccine trials so far is that most HIV-free volunteers who participate in HIV vaccine studies will apparently test positive for HIV for life. These individuals are known as vaccine-induced HIV positives, which, according to researchers, means they look positive on paper but are negative for HIV. Is this a case when positive means negative? Only time will tell.

MALARIA

A malaria vaccine is being moved into a large phase III trial in response to positive results. The data from the phase II trial were published in the *New England Journal of Medicine,* December 11, 2008. The vaccine reduced the incidence of the disease in children in Kenya and Tanzania by 53 percent over eight months. This could be wonderful news for the thousands of children in the African countries who have feared this disease for years.

GENITAL HERPES

At the Interscience Conference on Antimicrobial Agents and Chemotherapy held in Toronto, Ontario, in September 2000, researchers announced they had tested a vaccine that helps prevent genital herpes. Genital herpes, a sexually transmitted disease, affects about forty-five million people aged twelve years and older in the United States.

The vaccine was tested in nearly three thousand people who were in a relationship with a person who had the disease. The investigators found that 3 percent of the people in the study developed genital herpes after receiving the vaccine compared with 11 percent of those who had received a placebo. Another 3 percent got the infection but did not develop any genital sores.

The researchers also discovered something else about the vaccine: It was only effective in women who had never had cold sores. They believe the reason the vaccine is effective in women and not men has to do with anatomy. The speculation is that the vaginal fluid contains antibody functions that act against the herpes virus. The findings of the study led one of the lead investigators, Dr. Spotswood Spruance of the University of Utah in Salt Lake City, to say that his preference would be to give the vaccine to girls aged ten to thirteen years. Again, like the HIV vaccine, a genital herpes vaccine could be in your child's future.

RESPIRATORY SYNCYTIAL VIRUS (RSV)

The National Institute of Allergy and Infectious Disease (NIAID) is developing an intranasal RSV vaccine. RSV is the most common cause of serious lower respiratory tract infections in infants and young children worldwide. In the United States, nearly all children become infected with RSV by age two. Seventy-five thousand to 125,000 are hospitalized yearly. Globally, 64 million are affected, and there are 160,000 deaths per year. High-risk premature and cardiopulmonary children account for half of all hospital admissions. This would replace the monthly shot of immune globulin that children receive now.

PAINLESS VACCINES

Every year, about twelve billion shots are given to people around the world. Naturally, not all of them are vaccines, but a shot is a shot and a needle, well, it hurts. Just ask any kid. Researchers have been working on needle-free delivery systems for vaccines and other medicine for years, and several are on the horizon. Not only will needle-free methods be pain-free, they will also eliminate the swelling and tenderness that often accompanies shots, as well as the risk of contamination from dirty or mishandled needles.

The Flu Mist vaccine is a nasal spray presently on the market. It is not recommended for all ages but it has been found to be 98 percent effective against the flu if the viruses match the flu viruses of the season.

Other needle-free approaches include:

- Adhesive skin patches, similar to those used to help people quit smoking. The patch will seep vaccine into the bloodstream. Flu and tetanus are the most likely candidates for the first vaccine skin patches.
- Time-release pills. Vaccines will be coated in biodegradable microspheres, microscopic "bubbles" that can be taken as a pill or a nasal spray. The slow-release microspheres may offer lifetime immunity in one dose, and thus eliminate the need for booster shots.
- Edible vaccines. Someday when we ask "What's for dinner?" the answer may be a vaccine-laced potato, carrot, soybean, or banana.

EDIBLE VACCINES

Because food vaccines will be genetically engineered, they will not contain whole, live viruses as measles and rubella vaccines do today. They will likely be more like the hepatitis B vaccine, which is genetically engineered and contains selected protein portions. Those who oppose genetically engineered foods, including edible vaccines, argue that the unknowns are too great. Will edible vaccines damage the DNA of those who eat them? Will governments put edible vaccines on the market and not tell consumers?

SUPER-VACCINE?

Researchers with the Children's Vaccine Initiative (CVI), an organization composed of private and government groups from around the world, are developing a genetically engineered "super-vaccine," which they hope to give to all children orally at birth. This super-vaccine, nicknamed the Holy Grail by the CDC and the CVI, reportedly will contain the DNA from more than twenty viruses, parasites, and bacteria that cause various childhood diseases. The DNA will enter the cells of infants, and over a period of several months, the vaccine will be released.

The scheduled "recipe" for the super-vaccine includes three viruses for pneumonia, two for AIDS, four for dengue hemorrhagic fever (a mosquito-borne illness found in the tropics and subtropics), several viruses and bacteria for diarrheal diseases, two parasites for malaria, six viruses and bacteria for meningitis, three viruses for polio, and one appropriate organism each for diphtheria, hepatitis, measles, schistosomiasis (a parasitic disease common in Africa and Asia), tuberculosis, typhoid fever, and pertussis. When will this recipe be served up? No one knows, but vaccine manufacturers are looking for $500 million from international governments for development to make it a reality.

OTHER FUTURE VACCINES

Of the hundreds of vaccines on the drawing table and in trials, here are a few that you may see in a few years.

• **Cytomegalovirus vaccine:** The cytomegalic virus (CMV) causes a severe infection. Most people are exposed to this virus and some experience some minor respiratory symptoms from it, although some people have no symptoms at all. This virus is no problem for most people except for pregnant women and transplant patients. Pregnant women risk damaging the developing fetus (up to 15 percent will have permanent damage) if they get CMV during their first trimester. Transplant patients who have never had CMV but who receive a CMV-infected organ may develop a fatal illness. Twelve-year-old children are being considered for this vaccine.

• **Ulcer vaccine:** There are twenty-two million cases of ulcers each year caused by the bacteria *Helicobacter pylori*. The ulcer vaccine under development may help prevent many of these. In October 2000, researchers at the University of Padua in Italy announced they had developed an ulcer vaccine that proved effective in animals and would be tested in humans next.

• **Cancer vaccine:** Scientists have developed vaccines to help treat cancers that are in the early stages. The vaccines under consideration stimulate the immune system to allow the body to reduce tumors and destroy cancer cells. Some of the vaccines under development include those for skin cancer (melanoma), as well as prostate, colon, stomach, cervical, ovarian, lung, and breast cancers.

• **Alzheimer's disease vaccine:** At the World Alzheimer's Congress in July 2000, the Elan Corporation, an Irish pharmaceutical company that has developed an Alzheimer's vaccine, announced that its first human trials had been very successful. Dr. Ivan Lieberburg, executive vice president and chief science and medical officer for the company, said, "Assuming everything works out, this vaccine not only will treat Alzheimer's disease, but will also prevent Alzheimer's. It will completely change the face of Alzheimer's therapeutics now and forever if it works." Several other research teams are pursuing an Alzheimer's vaccine as well. The basic idea of the vaccines is to attack the plaques ("scars" composed of protein and other materials that build up) in the brain, which are a characteristic of the disease and are believed to be the cause of Alzheimer's. The outcome of these studies should also reveal whether plaques are truly the cause of Alzheimer's disease, which affects about four million Americans.

• **Chlamydia vaccine:** This sexually transmitted bacterial disease causes genital infections, including pelvic inflammatory disease. It may cause infertility if it spreads to the fallopian tubes. Chlamydia infects about 10 percent of sexually active women. A vaccine for this disease may be recommended for all twelve-year-olds.

BOTTOM LINE

Dozens, if not hundreds, of vaccines are just around the corner. This chapter has touched on just a few of those new possibilities. All of us need to watch how these new vaccines develop and be mindful of the ethical guidelines that need to develop along with them. We also certainly must be vigilant about our rights as parents concerning the administration of these vaccines. In the next part of this book, we look at the laws and parents' rights concerning vaccines. It is important that we see where these laws and rights are now, where they need to be modified, and how we can change them if we are to be faced with many more vaccines in the near future.

NOTES

Aviron press release. "Aviron Strengthens FluMist™ Commercial Infrastructure with Two Transactions in United Kingdom." Released October 11, 2000.

CNN release. "Alzheimer's Vaccine Seen as Treatment, Not Cure." At www.cnn.com/HEALTH/9907/08/alzheimers.vaccine.01.

Elliott, V. "Malaria Vaccine Proving Promising." *American Medical News* 52, no. 1 (January 5, 2009).

Halsey, Neal. Cited in Barbara Loe Fisher, "Shots in the Dark." *The Next City* (summer 1999): 52.

Schrof, Joannie M. "Miracle Vaccines." *U.S. News & World Report* (November 23, 1998).

Scientific American Web site: www.sciam.com/2000/0900issue/0900langridge.html.

Spruance, Spotswood. Retrieved from Reuters Health at http://thriveonline.oxygen.com/news/2000Sep18/27.html.

Sutton, P., and A. Lee. "Helicobactor Pylori Vaccines: The Current Status." *Alimentary Pharmacology and Therapeutics* 14, no. 9 (2000): 1107–18.

Tacket, C. O., et al. "Human Immune Responses to a Novel Norwalk Virus Vaccine Delivered in Transgenic Potatoes." *Journal of Infectious Diseases* 182, no. 1 (July 2000): 302–5.

Terence, Chea. "Novavax Wins $1 Mil to Make HPV Vaccine." *Washington Post* (October 10, 2000).

Walmsley, A. M., and C. J. Arntzen. "Plants for Delivery of Edible Vaccines." *Current Opinion on Biotechnology* 11, no. 2 (April 2000): 126–29.

www.cdc.gov/vaccines/program/iis/stds/cvx.htm.

Part III

TOOLS FOR PARENTS

Chapter 20

❋

Parents, the Law, and Insurance Companies

THE WORLD OF VACCINES IS AN UNCERTAIN ONE, AND UNCERtainty is something parents don't want to hear when it comes to determining their children's health. Although we all know there's nothing absolutely "for sure" in this world, knowing that a vaccine may cause serious complications or death is cause for parents to do a bit of investigating before they allow a needle to be jabbed into their child's arm.

That's why this chapter focuses on certainties: rights, rules, and laws concerning vaccinations. It explains your rights as parents when it comes to vaccinating your child, what exemptions you can seek, what laws protect your child concerning vaccine-related injuries, and how some of the vaccine laws work for and against your children.

PARENTS' RIGHTS: DO YOU HAVE ANY?

What are your rights when it comes to vaccinations? Should parents have the right to exempt their children from receiving vaccines that federal and state governments have mandated as necessary for public safety? Does it worry you that the government can mandate which vaccines your child must receive to enter day care or the school system? Do you wonder how far the government will go with that mandate?

These are hotly debated issues, especially as parents and medical professionals learn more about the possible adverse effects of vaccines, the questionable testing procedures that have been done, the conflicts of interest surrounding the people who are making decisions about which vaccines children receive, and the lack of research regarding the injuries and deaths that appear to be associated with vaccines. It's a debate that pits advocates for choice on one side and champions for public health on the other.

Rights in Jeopardy: Strong-Arm Tactics

As the number of parents who question the safety and effectiveness of vaccines grows, so do the reports of strong-arm tactics to prevent them from exercising their rights. Some states, for example, withhold a portion of a mother's welfare check if she does not have her children vaccinated. Individuals enrolled in the federal WIC (Women, Infants, and Children) program, which provides food to needy women and children, can also be denied food if they refuse vaccinations. Several states withhold $25 per child per month in state health aid for each child who has not received all the mandated vaccinations.

Jane Orient, M.D., executive director of the Association of American Physicians and Surgeons, says that she has heard reports of doctors who have threatened to remove children from their parents and have them placed with Child Protective Services if the parents refuse to have their child vaccinated. Children are not allowed to enter school or day care if they have not completed the required vaccination schedule (unless an exemption is sought—see chapter 21), and unvaccinated or partially vaccinated children are being kicked out of schools. Some congressional members have even suggested that federal income tax exemptions be denied parents who do not vaccinate their children.

Paul Offit, M.D., chief of infectious diseases at Children's Hospital of Philadelphia, believes "it is no more your right to catch and transmit a potentially fatal illness than it is your right to run a red light." He does not believe parents should be able to get exemptions because, he says, it places both their children and others at risk of disease. Might it be different if he had a child affected for life because of a serious side effect of a vaccine? If the vaccines really do as he believes they do and we have herd immunity, an occasional unvaccinated child should pose no threat to the vaccinated masses.

Clearly the issue of what parents' rights are when it comes to vaccinations could be a book of its own. The controversy and debates will continue. Parents can become active about the issue or monitor its progress by contacting the organizations listed in the appendix.

Strong-arm tactics are not just reserved for children and their parents. You may remember hearing stories about the anthrax vaccine, which all military personnel are required to receive. Hundreds of men and women in the armed forces have refused the controversial vaccine, and instead have chosen early retirement or court-martial.

In November 2007, parents of more than twenty-three hundred students in Prince George County, Maryland, who failed to get all of the mandated vaccinations were facing fines of $50 per day and up to ten days in jail if their children were not brought up to date on the required vaccinations. The parents were asked to appear in court and to have the vaccines administered by the courthouse. This was a first in the battle to get children fully vaccinated.

Subsequently, in 2008, New Jersey mandated flu vaccine and pneumococcal vaccine for preschoolers and the meningococcal and diphtheria-pertussis-tetanus vaccines for sixth graders. This was the first state in the country to mandate these vaccines for children of these ages.

Texas Governor Rick Perry attempted to mandate human papilloma virus vaccine for young girls in 2007 but met with tremendous opposition from parents and professionals.

Quiet Persuasion

Not all the persuasion to comply with mass immunization policies comes from government agencies and vaccine manufacturers, at least not directly. Nonprofit organizations such as Every Child By Two, which was founded by former First Lady Rosalyn Carter and Betty Bumpers, wife of Arkansas Senator Dale Bumpers, is credited with achieving passage of the laws requiring vaccinations for entry into school. Every Child By Two also promotes immunization registries (see "Vaccine Registry," below) and sends out notices to families to remind them when vaccines are due.

Few people can doubt that the founders of Every Child By Two and the vast majority of people who work for them have children's best interests in mind. But it should be known that this nonprofit is funded by the largest vaccine manufacturers in the United States—as well as the Centers for Disease Control (CDC). Another nonprofit organization, the CDC Foundation, established in 1995, uses its funds to help the CDC's effort to enforce mass vaccinations.

EXEMPTIONS:
YOUR RIGHT TO REFUSE VACCINES

Even though all states require children to receive specific vaccines before they can attend school, every state also allows at least one exemption, and many offer two and even three to that mandate. Yet most parents seem to know little or nothing about this option. If they ask their doctors or other vaccine providers about their state's exemption policies, the information is often given to them reluctantly or in such a way that it discourages parents from pursuing their rights. In fact, less than 2 percent of students across the United States take any type of exemption.

There are three types of exemptions from routine vaccination requirements: medical, philosophical, and religious. States can change their requirements at any time for any one or all of the exemptions, so I recommend you check with your state department of public health for the most recent regulations (see chapter 21).

Medical Exemption

Since January 1998, all fifty states have allowed medical exemptions from vaccinations required for entry into school. Parents who seek this exemption must provide the school with documentation from a licensed physician (a medical doctor or a doctor of osteopathy) or from a local board of health that explains why giving the vaccine would be detrimental to the child. Some of the medical reasons used for an exemption are explained below.

- **Vaccine reactions:** A child who has a severe allergic reaction (for example, shock, difficulty breathing, hives) or other immune or brain problems after receiving a vaccine should not get that vaccine again. The reaction may be to one of the ingredients in the vaccine or to the vaccine itself.

- **Weakened immune system:** People who are taking certain medications or who have certain illnesses should not receive live vaccines (such as varicella and MMR) because their immune system may not be able to fight off the virus. Drugs that weaken the immune system include steroids (except those that are used topically or inhaled, or if they have been used for less than fourteen days or every other day) and those used to treat cancer. People who have cancer, AIDS, or an inborn immune system weakness such as congenital immuno-deficiency—or who are receiving radiation treatments—should not get live vaccines.

- **Recipient of blood products:** Anyone who has received a blood transfusion or another blood product that contains antibodies should not get a live vaccine. The antibodies in the blood products can make the vaccine viruses inactive.

- **Proof of immunity:** Some states allow an exemption if you can produce proof that the child (or you) has immunity. It is necessary to check with your state's laws to determine if you have this option, and if so, which vaccines can be exempted with proof of immunity. To provide proof of immunity, you will need to have a blood test to measure the level of antibodies you have for the specific disease. If the antibody levels meet the standards set for the disease, you have proof of immunity.

In addition, many people, including researchers, parents, and health care providers, believe that some people have a genetic predisposition to experience negative reactions to certain vaccines. Such genetic tendencies may run in families and certain populations and are believed to be one reason some children develop conditions such as autism, diabetes, Crohn's disease, arthritis, and learning disorders after being vaccinated.

Benjamin Schwartz, acting director of epidemiology and surveillance for the Centers for Disease Control and Prevention's National Immunization Program, says there are no good data to support a genetic tendency for some people to experience adverse reactions to vaccines.

Unfortunately, vaccine providers do not screen for people who may have a family history of or predisposition for these disorders. This area deserves much more research.

Religious Exemption

The right to seek a religious exemption for vaccination is granted based on the right to freely exercise your religion, stated in the First Amendment to the Constitution. All states except Mississippi and West Virginia allow individuals to seek a religious exemption to vaccination. That does not mean that the other forty-eight states all interpret *religious exemption* in the same way. For example, in some states, those seeking a religious exemption must show they are members of a bona fide religion that specifically prohibits the use of invasive medical procedures such as vaccinations. One such religion is Christian Science, or the First Church of Christ Scientist.

Some states require a notarized waiver signed by the parents of the child, while others ask for a signed affidavit from the pastor of the church. In some states, a religious exemption is defined more loosely and is similar to a person's philosophical beliefs.

Because each state has different interpretations of what constitutes a religious exemption, you need to get a copy of your state's public health codes from the department of public health (see chapter 21) before you go forward.

State's health officials often challenge people who seek this exemption. Therefore, people who seek a religious exemption should be prepared to defend their position. It is not necessary in all states to belong to a church that specifically bans vaccinations in order to get an exemption; exemptions have been granted to parents of many different faiths and personal religious beliefs.

To support your defense, it is helpful to get a statement from a pastor, priest, rabbi, or other spiritual adviser attesting to your sincere religious beliefs, which you can submit along with your own written explanation of why you want the exemption. The state, if it decides to challenge you, must present "compelling State interest" to take away your right. The best argument a state has is to convince the court that failing to vaccinate a child poses a definite threat of spreading communicable disease and thus places the welfare of society at risk.

Philosophical Exemption

In 1990, a total of twenty-two states allowed philosophical exemptions. A decade later, the number had dropped to eighteen. At the time this book was published, those states were Arizona, Arkansas, California, Colorado, Idaho, Louisiana, Maine, Michigan, Minnesota, New Mexico, North Dakota, Ohio, Oklahoma, Texas, Utah, Vermont, Washington, and Wisconsin. In Arizona, the exemption applies only to elementary and middle school children; Nebraska and Missouri allow them for children in day care, and Missouri also permits them for children in Head Start programs.

The decline is the result of several state legislatures succumbing to pressure from their state departments of health, whose immunization departments are funded and/or staffed by the CDC, to drop the provision from their state code. In some states, citizens' groups have opposed deleting the exemption provision, and they have won. In others, a lack of organized opposition allowed the provision to be eliminated.

The requirements for getting a philosophical exemption differ from state to state. Generally, parents must provide a signed document that explains their philosophical objection to the vaccination. Such a document must be submitted every year in some states, while others allow the statement to apply for all of a child's school years.

LAW OR RECOMMENDATION: WHAT'S THE DIFFERENCE?

If the CDC recommends that all children receive the MMR vaccine, does that mean it is required by law in your state? Or does your state only require that measles and rubella vaccines be given?

There is a difference between what federal agencies or vaccine policy makers such as the American Academy of Pediatrics *recommend* and what your particular state *requires by law.* Before your child gets a vaccine or you get one, you may want to check to see what the vaccination laws are in your state. For example, although all states require that children get vaccines for diphtheria, several do not require pertussis, and two do not require tetanus. Therefore, you may have the option of choosing only one or two components of the MMR or DTP vaccine to meet your state's vaccine law requirements. (Naturally, you may still exercise your exemption rights if you so choose.)

ADVERSE REACTIONS TO VACCINES:
WHAT THE LAW SAYS

Under federal law, doctors and other health care professionals who administer vaccines are required to follow guidelines concerning how they give vaccines, required documentation, and the reporting of adverse reactions. It is important that you know what is required of those who administer vaccines, because these mandates ultimately protect you. These requirements include:

• **Reporting adverse events:** Any injuries, hospitalization, or death that occurs within thirty days of vaccination must be reported to the Vaccine Adverse Events Reporting System (VAERS; see chapter 22). The types of health problems to be reported include but are not limited to convulsions, coma, shock, paralysis, and other serious events. The National Childhood Vaccine Injury Compensation Act requires health care providers to report two types of events: any that are listed in the Reportable Events Table (the latest of which can be seen at http://bhpr.hrsa.gov/vicp/table.htm) that occur within the stated time frame, and any adverse events listed by the manufacturer as a contraindication to additional doses of the vaccine. The law states that those who administer vaccines have an obligation to report these events without passing judgment as to whether or not they believe the event was caused by the vaccine.

  Note: If your doctor or other health professional refuses or fails to report a serious adverse event to VAERS within thirty days regarding a vaccine you or your child has received, you can report the adverse reaction yourself (see chapter 22 for information).

• **Recording adverse reactions:** Doctors are required to

record any serious health problems following vaccination in a patient's permanent medical record.

- **Keeping permanent records:** The manufacturer, lot number, and date of all vaccines must be kept as part of a doctor's permanent records.
- **Providing information:** Before a health care professional administers a vaccine that is covered by the National Childhood Vaccine Injury Compensation Program, he or she must provide the patient or the patient's parent or guardian with information about the vaccine's risks and benefits. The CDC has created Vaccine Information Statements, or VIS, for this purpose. Your vaccine provider is required to give you a VIS for each vaccine administered and for each dose of the vaccine given. As mentioned earlier in the book, you should get the VIS and information from the vaccine's manufacturer from your doctor at a visit before the one at which the shots will be given. This will allow you time to read over the materials. You do have the right to ask for them and are encouraged to do so.

You should note that although vaccine providers are required by law to report only certain types of reactions, you as a parent or guardian of a child can report to VAERS any significant reaction that occurs after the administration of any vaccine that is licensed in the United States. See chapter 22 for information on how to file.

VACCINE INJURY COMPENSATION: WHAT THE LAW SAYS

In 1986, the US Congress enacted the National Childhood Vaccine Injury Compensation Act, which created the National Childhood

Vaccine Injury Compensation Program (NCVICP) and instituted the vaccine adverse event reporting and recording requirements. The NCVICP was created to provide compensation for injuries or death associated with receiving recommended childhood vaccinations. But this program did not come about easily.

The National Childhood Vaccine Injury Compensation Program

The National Childhood Vaccine Injury Compensation Program was born in response to the rising number of serious adverse reactions associated with the whole-cell pertussis portion of the DTP vaccine that had been administered in the United States since the 1950s (see chapter 7). By the mid-1980s, at least three hundred lawsuits had been filed against the vaccine manufacturers, and the number continued to rise. In response to the lawsuits, one of the three DTP producers stopped making the vaccine, and the other two found it very difficult to buy liability insurance. If the United States wanted to continue giving the DTP vaccine, something needed to be done.

The US manufacturers asked Congress to limit their liability and protect them from vaccine injury lawsuits not only for the DTP vaccine, but also for MMR and polio vaccines. At the same time, members of the NVIC wanted legislation that would protect the rights of families and enact vaccine safety reforms that would help prevent further vaccine injuries. Federal health officials and manufacturers still insisted that the vaccines were safe and that the children who had been injured or who had died had suffered through no fault of the vaccines.

But the NVIC scored a victory when, in 1986, President Ronald Reagan signed the National Childhood Vaccine Injury Compensation Act into law. This acknowledged that vaccines can harm and kill and created a federal compensation program by which vaccine-injured children and their families can receive financial help. However, the manufacturers also scored a victory in that they are protected from being sued in vaccine injury lawsuits.

The act also has other features:

- It protects the pediatricians, other health care providers, and vaccine manufacturers from any liability.
- There is a centralized reporting system, run by the FDA and CDC, which is used to monitor adverse reactions to vaccines.
- It mandates that parents must get vaccine benefit and risk information from doctors before vaccination and doctors must report and record vaccine adverse events.
- It helps ensure the vaccine supply and that routine mass immunizations will continue as required by the states.
- It requires periodic independent evaluations of any scientific evidence on adverse reactions to vaccinations.

If you or your child have been harmed because of routine vaccinations and the injuries have resulted in permanent damage, death, or medical expenses in excess of $1,000 (not reimbursed by insurance); or have lasted for more than six months, you have the right to seek compensation through the NCVICP. A description of the types of injuries covered under the program, as well as information on how to apply for compensation and the process that must be followed, is detailed in chapter 21.

Program Changes

Since 1995, it has been increasingly difficult for families to get compensation from the program. That's because in 1995,

Department of Health and Human Services (DHHS) Secretary Donna Shalala and other federal health officials toughened the guidelines under which compensation would be considered. Although Shalala added a few injuries to the list, she also deleted some that historically had been associated with many more claims than the ones she added. The General Accounting Office noted that it would probably be harder for most parents to get compensation with the new guidelines.

And that appears to be true. As of 2000 three out of four vaccine-injured children were being refused financial assistance, even though more than $1 billion was available in the trust fund for this purpose. (The money comes from a surcharge placed on each vaccine given.)

Another problem is that the legal process has become so complex that it can take up to nine years for cases to be resolved. Clifford J. Shoemaker, an attorney who has represented vaccine victims for more than twenty years, believes Shalala's changes "effectively devastated the program." But the program's director, Thomas E. Balbier Jr., claims that Shalala's modifications simply brought the list of injuries that are accepted for compensation "in line with science."

The families of the autistic children have had a difficult time having their cases heard in the vaccine court. After the statement by the Institute of Medicine in 2004 claiming no connection causally between vaccines and autism, it has been an uphill battle for them. In 2008, however, with the settlement of the Hannah Poling case, the door to the court has opened a little wider for these children and their parents. The years following that decision will decide the fate of these families as far as receiving any compensation for medical care for the children.

VACCINE LAWS: A BRIEF HISTORY

In 1905, a Mr. Jacobson, who lived in Cambridge, Massachusetts, violated a 1902 Cambridge Board of Health mandate that required all city residents to be vaccinated for smallpox. Mr. Jacobson told the court that he had "suffered seriously from previous vaccination," and so he refused to be vaccinated again. Such a refusal, when made by anyone older than twenty-one years of age, carried a fine of $5.

Mr. Jacobson's case made it to the Supreme Court, where the court affirmed the right of any state legislature to enforce mandatory vaccinations. In *Jacobson v. Massachusetts,* the court stated that "in a free country, where the government is by the people . . . what the people believe is for the common welfare must be accepted as tending to promote the common welfare whether it does in fact or not." It also said that "the interests of the many [should not be] subordinated to the wishes or convenience of the few." Mr. Jacobson was the few; he lost the case and $5.

This case was perhaps a harbinger of things to come. In 1904, thirteen of the then forty-five states excluded unvaccinated children from public schools. Of course back then there was only one vaccine, for smallpox. In the intervening years, vaccines for diphtheria, tetanus, and pertussis were developed, but it wasn't until the Sabin live oral polio vaccine was introduced in 1960 that there was an increased interest in making vaccinations mandatory for school admission. President John F. Kennedy helped kick off the flurry by submitting the Vaccination Assistance Act of 1962, which provided federal moneys and CDC personnel to local health departments and states to encourage vaccinations. This act was largely responsible for getting all the states to quickly incorporate federal vaccine recommendations into state law.

Today federal vaccination policies trickle down to the state level from two committees: the FDA's Vaccines and Related Biological Products Advisory Committee (VRBPAC), which determines whether new vaccines are effective and safe; and the CDC's Advisory Committee on Immunization Practices (ACIP), which recommends which vaccines should be on the Childhood Immunization Schedule. It is interesting to note that physicians who sit on that committee may legally own patents on vaccines. The American Academy of Pediatrics (AAP), a private organization representing pediatricians, also makes vaccine policy recommendations that conform to CDC guidelines. The CDC and AAP Schedule is the one most states adopt and require of children if they are to be allowed to enter school, and day care in some cases. There are slight variations among the states (for example, not all states require the varicella vaccine, and some don't require all three components of the MMR vaccine), but basically the requirements for all states are similar.

VACCINE REGISTRY

In 1995, DHHS Secretary Donna Shalala laid the groundwork for a centralized database that will contain the medical records of every child in the United States. She gave the Social Security Administration the right to reveal the Social Security number of newborn infants to state health department officials for use in their vaccine tracking registry. Shalala's move allows the DHHS to disclose information about individuals without their consent if it is for the purpose of administering a government-run public health program or for medical research.

The plan links all of the states into one network. This network will be able to track which parents have or have not vaccinated their children. To help states establish a vaccine tracking system and enforce their vaccination mandates, each state is eligible for federal grants. In addition, they also get moneys from pharmaceutical companies, specifically vaccine manufacturers. The Robert Wood Johnson Foundation (Johnson & Johnson, which funds the vaccine program All Kids Count) is one such funding company. Its vaccine ties are with Merck & Company, which manufactures MMR, varicella, and hepatitis B vaccines. In 1989, Merck joined with Johnson & Johnson to form Worldwide Consumer Pharmaceuticals Company.

Dangers of a National Registry

With the electronic surveillance program in place, the government will be allowed to deny more citizens their rights if it believes the citizens are not following certain health policies in the interest of public safety. This is especially frightening given the fact that there are hundreds of vaccines under development, some of which may be mandated by the government in the future. I believe that this medical registry erodes privacy, medical freedom, and the right to self-determination.

Goal: Vaccinate the World

In 1993, DHHS Secretary Donna Shalala was given the authority by Congress to reward states between $50 and $100 for each fully immunized child. This plan was reinforced in 1994 when the DHHS published the National Vaccine Plan (NVP), whose goal is to vaccinate every American child with every current and future government-recommended vaccine. The NVP is actually part of the larger Children's Vaccine Initiative (CVI), which was founded in 1990 in New York City at the World Summit for Children. The initiative, which is funded by the World Bank, the World Health Organization, the United Nation's Children's Fund (UNICEF), and other organizations, has as its goal to vaccinate all the children of the world with existing and future vaccines.

VACCINES AND INSURANCE: WHO PAYS?

Most insurance plans, including HMOs, pay for required childhood vaccines. However, parents should check with their individual insurance providers before making that assumption. For vaccines that are not required or if you request a mercury-free vaccine that your doctor must special-order, check with your insurance provider. There is also a Web site that provides information on insurance companies' policies on vaccine coverage as well as trends in the field: www.insure.com.

To ensure that uninsured children would still get their required vaccines, the Vaccines for Children (VFC) program was established by the government in 1993. The program provides free vaccines to children who are defined as "federally vaccine eligible" (both uninsured and Medicaid-eligible children). Other children also eligible under the VFC program are Native Americans, Alaskan Native children, and children whose insurance does not pay for immunizations. Eligible children must be eighteen years of age or younger. The VFC program covers all six of the vaccines recommended by the Advisory Committee on Immunization Practices.

BOTTOM LINE

At the National Vaccine Information Center Conference on Vaccination in September 2000, Barbara Loe Fisher said, "If the state can track down and force individuals against their will to be injected with biologicals of unknown toxicity today, will there be any limit on what freedoms that government can take away in the name of the greater good tomorrow?" Fisher's words remind us that unless we are prepared to stand up for our rights, they can be taken away. Parents cannot afford to be like those in the states that lost their philosophical exemption because of lack of protest by their citizens. We need to be aware of the laws concerning vaccines and be prepared to challenge them if we do not believe they are in the best interests of our children.

NOTES

Centers for Disease Control and Prevention. Vaccine Information Statements. May 4, 2000.

Health Services and Resources Administration Web site: www.hcfa.gov/init/chivfc.htm.

Hernandez, Nelson. "Get Kids Vaccinated or Else, Parents Told." *Washington Post.* http://tinyurl.com/2jevda.

Koch, Kathy. "Vaccine Controversies." *CQ Researcher* 10, no. 28 (August 25, 2000): 641–72.

National Vaccine Information Center Web site: www.nvic.org.

Richardson, Dawn. "Summary of the 9/28/99 Congressional Hearing on Vaccine Injury Compensation Program." At www.planetchiropractic.com/vaccine.htm.

Schafer Autism Report 11, no. 176.1 (December 11, 2007).

Severyn, K. M. "Mandatory Vaccination." Presentation at the 56th Annual Meeting of the Association of American Physicians and Surgeons, October 14, 1999. At www.all.org/activism/pox02.htm.

Vaccine Information Center, Sherri Tenpenny, DO: www.drtenpenny.com.

Chapter 21

❖

What You Can Do to Ensure
Your Child's Safety

EVERY JOURNEY BEGINS WITH THE FIRST STEP. YOU HAVE already taken that step by reading this book and learning more about vaccines and how they may affect your child and you. You've read about the benefits and the risks, the knowns and unknowns, and what the future may hold. You've learned that there are organizations you can contact to help you learn more about vaccines and those that can help you if your child becomes injured because of a vaccine. You've learned that there is much more to vaccines than a simple shot in the arm, a few tears, and a Band-Aid. And you've learned that you have the right and the power to make sure your child is as safe as possible when it comes time to consider immunizations.

This chapter brings together some tools for you to take action to protect your children and yourself against possible dangers associated with vaccinations. When you use the guidelines and suggestions in this chapter, you will join your voice with those of other concerned parents around the world.

HOW TO REDUCE REACTIONS TO VACCINATIONS

Taking your infant or young child in to the doctor for his or her vaccinations can be scary for both you and the child. The goal should be to make the experience before, during, and after as pain- and trauma-free as possible. Here are some tips:

- Your child should be examined before every vaccination to make sure he or she is in good health, and especially does not have a fever. The results of the examination should be noted in your child's medical records.
- Ask your doctor which vaccine your child will get at his or her next visit and request the Vaccine Information Statement (VIS) information and the vaccine package insert so you will have time to learn about the vaccine before it is given.
- Tell your doctor if your child has been ill recently or if anyone in the child's family is currently ill. Evidence indicates that individuals who have a viral or bacterial infection may not mount an adequate antibody response to the vaccine, plus they are at increased risk of having adverse reactions.
- Before you go to the health care provider who will be administering the vaccine, write down a complete family and personal medical history for your child to give to the doctor. This includes information on any family member, including grandparents, cousins, uncles, aunts, and siblings, who has a history of seizures, adverse reactions to vaccinations, autoimmune disease, neurologic disease, or severe allergies. This information should be in your child's medical files.

- Make sure the injection is being given in the correct part of the body and in the correct manner. How and where injections are made have an impact on the amount of pain, redness, and swelling that may occur at the site. Vaccines should never be injected into the buttocks, because there is a chance of injuring a large nerve that crosses through this body area. Proper administration of vaccines is also important because those that are given incorrectly may not be effective and will need to be repeated.
- Ask to see the package insert that accompanied the vaccine to make sure it is the vaccine you agreed upon with the doctor. You should ask for a copy of your child's vaccination records for your own personal files. That record should include the name of the vaccines, the dates given, and the lot numbers. If the lot numbers are not included on your copy, ask for them.
- One way to reduce the pain of the injection is to apply firm pressure to the site immediately before and after the shot is given.
- Distraction from the actual shot works for some children. Bring along a toy, or video game for older children.
- Ibuprofen can help relieve pain, swelling, and tenderness. A low fever is not usually a problem and doesn't need medication. If the child's temperature goes above 100.6 degrees for twenty-four hours or more, call your physician.
- Acetaminophen may help prevent seizures in children who have a tendency for them when they have a fever.
- Fruit juice before and after the DTaP shot can help to maintain blood sugar levels.
- An ice bag or cold compress on the injection site can reduce swelling and pain.
- I give vitamin A in the form of cod liver oil at the Daily Recommended Intake for age. This is about 1,250 to 5,000

IU per day depending on the child's age and weight. For many brands, 1,250 IU equals half a teaspoon; however, follow the instructions on individual brands, as they are not all the same. If your child is taking a multiple vitamin-mineral supplement, make sure you allow for the amount of vitamin A in the supplement before giving cod liver oil, as you do not want to give too high a dosage. The total amount of vitamin A from all supplements given in one day should not exceed the Daily Recommended Intake.

- Vitamin C protects against adverse reactions. On the day of the shots and the day after, I recommend 150 mg liquid twice daily to infants. Follow package directions for measurement instructions. For toddlers, consider giving 300 mg twice daily in either liquid or children's vitamin C tablets.

- Vaccines that come in single-dose vials are preferred over multidose vials because the potency of the vaccine is known, and single-dose vials are mercury-free. If your child's vaccine is being drawn from a multidose vial, make sure the nurse or doctor shakes the vial before she or he draws out the vaccine so the contents are more evenly distributed. Check the package insert and do not let anyone give your child a vaccine with thimerosal in the ingredient list.

- A sensible, healthy diet is recommended at all times to help keep the immune system operating at its best.

KNOW YOUR STATE'S LAWS ON VACCINATIONS

Each state has different legal requirements concerning vaccines and admittance to school, and these laws can change frequently. There are several ways you can get information about your state's laws on vaccinations:

- Contact the department of public health in your state and ask that a copy be sent to you.
- Ask your public librarian to help you locate the public health codes and education and welfare laws that describe vaccination requirements for school entry in your state.
- Visit your library and ask for a copy of the State Statute Revised Law Book. Look under the Public Health Law or the Communicable Disease section.
- Contact your state representative and ask for a copy.
- If you become a member of the National Vaccine Information Center (NVIC; see the appendix), a summary of your state's vaccination law may be available to you.

The sources listed above are the most reliable. Do not depend on information given to you by a friend, nurse, or school principal. Even your doctor or other health care professionals may not always have the most up-to-date information. Although they may believe they have the correct or most recent information, they often do not.

QUESTIONS TO ASK THE DOCTOR BEFORE VACCINATING YOUR CHILD

All health care providers who give mandated vaccines are required by law to give the parents or legal caregivers of the child—or adults if they are the recipients of a vaccine—a Vaccine Information Statement. The VIS is an information sheet produced by the Centers for Disease Control and Prevention that explains the benefits and risks of a vaccine. The National Childhood Vaccine Injury Act of 1986 required that a VIS be given to all parents or legal representatives for many of the vaccines. You are strongly encouraged to ask for a VIS for any vaccine if your provider does not offer it. You can also get a current VIS on the Internet at the National Immunization Program Web site (www.cdc.gov/nip) and the Immunization Action Coalition Web site (www.immunize.org).

The VIS answers some questions you may have for your health care provider, but certainly not all of them. Ask your doctor these questions before your child receives any vaccine, and also ask for the product information that accompanies it.

- **What are the symptoms of a reaction to the vaccine?** You should know what symptoms may occur, how long it usually takes for them to appear (see the appropriate chapters for the symptoms for each individual vaccine), and when to seek medical attention. The VIS does not cover all this information completely.
- **Can I get mercury-free vaccines?** If the doctor says no, get a second opinion. There is at least one mercury- (thimerosal-) free brand for every required childhood vaccine on the market. If your doctor does not have the mercury-free vaccines, ask him or her to order them for you. (Contact the CDC at 800-232-2522 or at www.cdc.gov for the most up-to-date list.)
- **Which polio vaccine are you using?** In January 2000, the CDC recommended that the oral, live polio vaccine not be given to children, because the live virus can pass through the baby's stool and cause polio in either the child or the child's caregiver. Ask that only the inactive injected vaccine be given to your child for all four doses.

QUESTIONS TO ASK YOURSELF
BEFORE YOUR CHILD GETS VACCINATED

You know your child better than anyone, so it is important that you ask yourself the following questions before your child receives a vaccination. A yes answer to any of these questions may mean that your child should either not get the vaccine at all or that it should be delayed. Discuss any yes answers with your physician before the vaccine is given.

1. Is my child sick today? The general recommendation is that children who have a moderate or severe illness should postpone receiving the vaccine until they have recovered. You have the right to wait until children who have even a mild illness are well.

2. Does my child have any allergies to medications, food, or any vaccine?

3. Has my child ever had a reaction to a vaccine? I recommend that you discuss with your doctor any reactions your child may have had to past vaccinations to see if they may affect the decision to give your child another vaccine. Vitamin C may help protect against adverse reactions. On the day of the shots and the day after, I generally recommend 150 mg liquid twice daily to infants. Follow package directions for measurement instructions. For toddlers, give 300 mg twice daily in either liquid or children's vitamin C tablets.

4. Has my child taken cortisone, prednisone, other steroids, or anticancer drugs, or undergone X-ray treatment in the last three months? Has anyone who lives with or who takes care of my child had any of these treatments within the last three months?

5. Does my child or any person who lives with or cares for my child have cancer, AIDS, leukemia, or any other immune system disorder?

6. Is my child/teen pregnant or is there a chance she may become pregnant in the next three months?

7. Has my child ever had a seizure or a brain problem?

8. Has my child received a blood or plasma transfusion or been given immune (gamma) globulin within the past year?

When you visit your doctor, bring your child's vaccination record card with you. It is important that all your child's vaccinations be recorded on the card because you will need it as proof of vaccination when it is time for your child to enter day care and school.

MY VACCINATION RECOMMENDATIONS

The following are recommendations for vaccinations that I believe are safer for the general population: These are recommendations that I make to patients and to families of patients in my own practice. These suggestions are not meant to be a substitute for what your doctor recommends. It is important that all parents realize that regardless of which vaccination schedule they use, there is no way to guarantee that their children will not get any of the illnesses against which they are immunized. No vaccination schedule is foolproof, just as no two children are alike; each one has his or her own genetic susceptibilities, environmental influences, dietary needs, and lifestyles. In addition to the vaccination recommendations, I encourage all mothers to breast-feed their children for at least the first six months if possible, as this provides infants with the best chance to receive passive immunity from their mothers during this time. I also urge all breast-feeding mothers to eat a nutritious diet and take vitamin supplements while breast-feeding.

Hepatitis B

In my practice, I do not recommend the hepatitis B vaccine for the infant unless the mother is positive for hepatitis B. Those children will get the hepatitis B vaccine at birth as they have for years. If mothers who are hepatitis-B-negative make the decision to give their child the vaccine, the following steps may reduce side effects:

- For children attending day care, consider postponing the vaccines until just before starting day care if the state mandates the vaccine for entry.
- For children not attending day care, consider postponing the vaccine until sometime between five and twelve years. Give the second shot one month after the first shot and the third at least six months after the first.

The goal of these recommendations is to postpone the vaccine as long as possible—thus reducing the possibility of adverse reactions—while staying within the laws of your particular state.

Hib, IPV, DTaP (All Should Be Mercury-Free)

I generally start Hib at four months with IPV (polio), followed by the DTaP at five months. In this case I believe it is relatively safe to give two vaccines—Hib and IPV—together, as the polio vaccine is much less likely to cause reactions.

Second series at six months (Hib and IPV), followed by DTaP at seven months.

Third series at eight months (Hib), followed by DTaP at nine months.

Fourth series at seventeen months (Hib, IPV) and eighteen months for the DTaP.

Boosters for DTaP and IPV at four and five years of age. Tdap if titers are negative at twelve years of age.

Pneumococcal

Because the safety data are not clear, I do not recommend the Prevnar vaccine. There are findings to suggest that the eighty-three strains not covered by the vaccine may be getting stronger and more resistant to antibiotics. In my practice, I recommend that the adult pneumococcal vaccine, Pneumovax, be given at two. In the future, a nine- or eleven-valent pneumococcal vaccine would be a viable alternative for the younger child (seven to eighteen months).

Varicella

It is my practice not to give this vaccine to one-year-old children. I usually hold this vaccine until twelve years of age and give it only if the child does not test to be immune to chicken pox already. If the vaccine is given, a booster may be necessary so that the child does not get chicken pox as a young adult when the disease would be more serious.

MMR

I recommend that the measles, mumps, and rubella be split into three vaccines and given six months apart, starting at fifteen months with the single measles vaccine. The rubella could be given at twenty-one months and the mumps shot at twenty-seven months. It should not be necessary to booster these at preschool time, but a titer should be drawn to demonstrate immunity. If the child is only immune to one or two of the trio, those single vaccines could be given instead of the combination MMR. At the time of this writing, Merck has stopped making the single vaccines. The company has not made it clear if this will be a permanent policy. In fact, 2011 has been mentioned as a possible date to resume manufacture of the single vaccines. I tell parents to be patient and to call Merck to request that the single vaccines be manufactured again before deciding to give the MMR.

Influenza

In my practice, I do not recommend this for young children and pregnant women. Much of the supply still contains thimerosal, the ethyl-mercury-containing preservative.

Hepatitis A

This vaccine is not recommended for all children in my practice as a routine part of the schedule. I reserve it for those living in endemic areas or for those traveling to areas where the disease is endemic. The threat and severity of the disease do not outweigh the possible side effects of the vaccine preparation.

Rotavirus

Because the possible side effects of this vaccine are serious and the disease itself does not cause epidemic mortality, I do not recommend this as a routine part of my patient's early vaccine schedule.

Meningococcal

I feel that this vaccine can be held until adolescents are ready to attend college and live in a dorm unless there have been cases reported in the community. Extra precautions should be taken with adolescents from families with a history of autoimmune illnesses because of the risk for Guillain-Barré syndrome.

HPV

At this point, I do not recommend this vaccine for any of my patients—especially children under eighteen years of age. There are questions involving the safety profile that have not been resolved.

BOTTOM LINE: ACTIONS PARENTS CAN TAKE

- Be informed. Learn all you can about the risks and benefits of any vaccine you are considering. Do not be satisfied with information from only one side of the issue. In addition to getting information from your doctor and any literature he or she gives to you, explore some of the books and Internet sites listed in the back of this book. They provide a wealth of information and, in the case of the Internet, can keep you informed of the latest changes and research in the field of vaccines.
- Know your state's laws about which vaccines are required for school entrance or day care and which ones can be eliminated. Also, know your state's vaccination exemption laws.
- Ask for thimerosal-free vaccines.
- Because any illness weakens the immune system, I recommend that children who have even a mild illness not be vaccinated until they have recovered.

- If possible, do not allow your children to receive vaccines for more than four organisms in one day. For example, if the doctor suggests giving the hepatitis B, DTaP, Hib, and polio vaccines all on the same day, ask to come back for two of the vaccines during a later visit.
- If your state requires the MMR vaccine for school admittance and you wish your child to receive it, request that the individual vaccines for measles, mumps, and rubella be given separately, if available. I suggest the measles component at fifteen months, rubella at twenty-one months, and mumps at twenty-seven months. You have the right to ask for this, even though some doctors may resist. Some states do not require all three vaccines; check your state public health laws.
- Follow the suggestions on how to reduce reactions to vaccines explained in this chapter.
- Monitor your child for adverse reactions and report them immediately to your doctor.
- Report adverse reactions to VAERS yourself if your doctor refuses to do so.
- Do not allow your children to receive vaccines that contain ingredients to which they are allergic: yeast in hepatitis B, eggs in MMR, neomycin in MMR and varicella.
- Consider having the hepatitis B vaccine given when your children are older than four years unless they are in day care.
- If possible, postpone the varicella vaccine until your children are twelve years old if they do not have immunity to chicken pox.
- If possible, check MMR vaccine titers (antibody levels) before your children get booster shots at four to five years of age. If the antibody levels are high enough, the booster shots may not be necessary.
- You can help protect the child with vitamin A in the form of cod liver oil and with vitamin C as previously discussed.

Test titers for immunity before school, because it may be possible to avoid a booster dose.

- I still do not recommend that women receive the MMR vaccine before or while breast-feeding.

RECOMMENDED VACCINE SCHEDULE

Birth—Hepatitis B if the mother is Hepatitis-B positive
4 months—Hib, IPV
5 months—DTaP
6 months—Hib, IPV
7 months—DTaP
8 months—Hib
9 months—DTaP
15 months—Measles
17 months—Hib, IPV
18 months—DTaP
21 months—Rubella
24 months—Pneumovax
27 months—Mumps
4–5 years—DTaP, IPV
4–5 years—Hepatitis A if in endemic area
4–5 years—Test titers for M, M, and R; booster if negative
5–12 years—Hepatitis B, if required by law
12 years—Varicella if titer is negative
12 years—Tdap if titers are negative
On admission to college dorm—Meningococcal

*If the nine- or eleven-valent pneumococcal vaccine becomes available, it can be given at 6, 9, and 18 months. Pneumovax would not be given in this case at 24 months.

NOTES

Centers for Disease Control and Prevention Web site: www.cdc.gov/nip.

Fisher, Barbara Loe. *The Consumer's Guide to Childhood Vaccines.* Vienna, VA: National Vaccine Information Center, 1997, 47.

Miller, Neil Z. *Vaccines: Are They Really Safe and Effective?* Santa Fe, NM: New Atlantean Press, 2008.

National Vaccine Information Center: www.nvic.org.

Sears, Robert. *The Vaccine Book: Making the Right Decision for Your Child,* New York, NY: Hachette Book Group, 2007.

Chapter 22

❀

The Vaccine Adverse Events
Reporting System

THE VACCINE ADVERSE EVENTS REPORTING SYSTEM (VAERS) is a program sponsored by the Centers for Disease Control and Prevention (CDC) and the Food and Drug Administration (FDA). The purpose of VAERS is to detect possible indicators of adverse events associated with vaccinations. To properly validate the indicators from VAERS and to determine whether there is a cause-and-effect relationship between a vaccine and the reported event, scientific studies are nearly always required.

Both the FDA and CDC review the information that is submitted to VAERS: the FDA reviews individual reports to determine if the reported reaction is listed in the product labeling and monitors any trends of reports that come in from individual vaccine makers; the CDC focuses on the bigger picture, looking for trends and associations among reported events. You can obtain copies of their published reviews from VAERS (see the appendix for contact information).

REPORTS TO VAERS

Although anyone can file a report with VAERS, most reports are submitted by health care providers (private providers make up 16 percent of the total and state health departments 29 percent, for a total of 45 percent) and vaccine manufacturers (40 percent). Parents, patients, and guardians are responsible for only 3 percent of the reports filed. The remaining 12 percent of reports come from other or unknown sources.

Of all the adverse events reported to VAERS, approximately 85 percent are classified as mild and include fever, mild irritability, crying, injection site irritation, and other minor episodes. The remaining 15 percent involve serious and life-threatening reactions that have resulted in hospitalization, permanent disability, or death.

If you or your child has a moderate or severe health problem after a vaccination, it should be reported to VAERS by you, your doctor, or your state health department. You have the right to report any significant health problem that occurs after a vaccine has been given, even if you are not certain that the vaccine caused the reaction. If your doctor refuses to report, you can do so yourself. Every report that is sent to VAERS provides essential information that the FDA and CDC can analyze along with the tens of thousands of other reports they receive each year. The information you submit can help them develop safer vaccine procedures and hopefully reduce the risks associated with vaccinations.

INTERPRETING DATA FROM VAERS

The VAERS program encourages the reporting of any significant adverse event that occurs after vaccination and does not make a judgment as to whether the event is merely a coincidence or is truly a result of receiving a vaccine. Therefore, the fact that any given report has been filed with VAERS does not mean a vaccine has caused the health problem.

REPORTING A REACTION

VAERS has a special report form you can use to submit your information. There are several ways you can obtain a copy of this form:

- The *Physicians' Desk Reference* (*PDR*) has a sample copy. This reference book can be found in most libraries; ask your reference librarian.
- Call VAERS at 800-822-7967 for preaddressed postage-paid forms.
- Fax your request to the toll-free fax line at 877-721-0366.
- You can download a copy of the form from several different Web sites: the VAERS site at www.vaers.org; the FDA's site at www.fda.gov/cber/vaers/vaers.htm; or the CDC's site at www.cdc.gov/nip.

When you make your report, be as specific and complete as possible. The form asks for, among other things, which vaccine was given, its manufacturer and lot number, and whether the child had any reactions to previous vaccines. There is also a space for you to describe the reaction(s) in your own words, including symptoms and time course.

GETTING INFORMATION FROM VAERS

If you want to know if certain adverse reactions for specific vaccines have been reported to VAERS, you can request individual reports by sending a written request to:

Food and Drug Administration
Freedom of Information Staff (HFI-35)
5600 Fishers Lane
Rockville, MD 20857
301-443-2414 or fax 301-443-1726

VAERS will also provide consumers with data from its database, without revealing any personal information, for a nominal fee. Requests for information can be made to:

National Technical Information Service
5285 Port Royal Road
Springfield, VA 22161
703-487-4650

NATIONAL VACCINE INFORMATION CENTER
VACCINE REACTION REGISTRY

Since 1982, the nonprofit Vaccine Information Center has been operating a vaccine reaction registry to serve as a "check and balance" on the VAERS system. Vaccine reaction data is being collected to serve as a foundation for independent, non-governmental, non-industry scientific research to help prevent vaccine reactions. To report a vaccine reaction to NVIC, go to www.909shot.com.

VACCINE-RELATED INJURIES:
WHAT YOU CAN DO

Under the National Childhood Vaccine Injury Compensation Program (NCVICP), you can seek compensation if your child has been injured by routine vaccinations. There are very specific requirements you must meet to qualify for the program, as well as a certain process that must be followed. Both of these items are explained here.

The NCVICP Vaccine Injury Table

The NCVICP Vaccine Injury Table is a list of the types of injuries that are accepted under the National Childhood Vaccine Injury Compensation Program to be considered for compensation. The entries change periodically; to see the most up-to-date table, go to www.vaers.org. It includes many changes that were made since the program started, including but not limited to the addition of rotavirus as of October 22, 1998, and the addition of pneumococcal conjugate vaccine as of December 18, 1999. You can also call VAERS at 800-822-7967.

The Process

The NCVICP is overseen by three entities: the US Court of Federal Claims, the Department of Health and Human Services (DHHS), and the Department of Justice. The process for seeking compensation for harm allegedly suffered is as follows:

- You will probably want to consult with a lawyer who is familiar with vaccine-related compensation or an injury specialist.

- A petition for compensation is filed with the Court of Federal Claims.
- A physician from the DHHS, Division of Vaccine Injury Compensation, reviews the petition to see if it meets the requirements for compensation.
- An attorney from the Department of Justice represents the DHHS's position on the petition in hearings, which are held before a "special master." This is an attorney, appointed by the judges of the court, who makes the initial decision for or against compensation.
- You may appeal any decision against your claim to the court, then to the Federal Circuit Court of Appeals, or seek review by the Supreme Court.

These are the general guidelines for applying for compensation. For injuries or deaths that occurred before Ocober 1, 1988: If you did not file a claim for compensation by January 31, 1996, the statute of limitations has run out. However, you may pursue a lawsuit (for example, sue the vaccine manufacturer) without time restrictions.

For injuries or deaths that occurred *after* October 1, 1988, the following guidelines apply:

- You are required to apply for federal compensation before you can pursue a lawsuit.
- The program may offer to pay up to $250,000 for a vaccine-associated death.
- The program may offer to pay for all past and future unreimbursed (through insurance) medical expenses and nursing and custodial care; up to $250,000 for pain and suffering; and loss of earned income.
- If you turn down this offer or the program turns down your claim, you can then file a lawsuit.

- Claims for compensation must be filed within twenty-four months of a death and thirty-six months of an injury.

The Compensation System and How It Works, published by the National Vaccine Information Center, provides helpful information on how to file a claim, what to expect when you do, and how the judgments are made. The NVIC also maintains a directory of attorneys who are familiar with vaccine injury claims.

How to Make a Claim

To get an information packet that explains how to file a claim, the criteria for eligibility, and the documents you need to make a claim, you can call the National Childhood Vaccine Injury Compensation Program at 800-338-2382. You can also contact the program on the Internet at www.hrsa.gov/bhpr/vicp, or you can write to:

National Vaccine Injury Compensation Program
Parklawn Building, Room 8A-46
5600 Fishers Lane
Rockville, MD 20857

For information on the requirements for filing a petition and the rules of the US Court of Federal Claims, call the court at 202-219-9657, or write to:

US Court of Federal Claims
717 Madison Place, NW
Washington, DC 20005

NOTES

Centers for Disease Control and Prevention Web site: www.cdc.gov/nip.

Food and Drug Administration Web site: www.fda.gov/cber/vaers/vaers.htm.

Immunization Action Coalition Web site: www.immunize.org.

Kalokerinos, Archie. *Every Second Child*. New Canaan, CT: Keats Publishing, 1981.

National Immunization Program Web site: www.cdc.gov/nip.

National Vaccine Information Center Med Alerts: www.medalerts.org.

National Vaccine Information Center Web site: www.909shot.com.

Vaccination Adverse Events Reporting System Web site: www.vaers.org.

Appendix:
Organizations and Web Sites

MEDICAL ASSOCIATIONS AND RELATED
ORGANIZATIONS

For information about vaccinations, the diseases they are designed
to prevent, and complications associated with vaccine use, you can
contact the following organizations:

American Academy of Family Physicians
11400 Tomahawk Creek Parkway
Leawood, KS 66211-2672
Voice: 913-906-6000
Web: www.aafp.org
E-mail: fp@aafp.org
Provides information on vaccines and childhood health issues.

American Academy of Pediatrics
141 Northwest Point Boulevard
Elk Grove Village, IL 60007
Voice: 847-228-5005
Web: www.aap.org
E-mail: kidsdocs@aap.org
Provides news briefs, policy statements, and other information on
immunization and childhood health issues.

American Medical Association
515 North State Street
Chicago, IL 60610
Voice: 312-464-5000
Web: www.americanmedicalassociation.org
The Web site has a search feature and a patient information feature
  where you can get health information and physician referrals.

Association of Maternal and Child Health Programs
1220 19th Street, NW, Suite 801
Washington, DC 20036
Voice: 202-775-0436
Web: www.amchp1.org
E-mail: info@amchp.org
Mission: to promote and advance national and state policies and
  programs and lobby policy makers on maternal and child health
  needs.

Association of State and Territorial Health Officials
1275 K Street, NW, Suite 800
Washington, DC 20005-4006
Voice: 202-371-9090
Web: www.astho.org
Engages in legislative, educational, scientific, and program issues for
  activities concerning public health.

Autism Research Institute
4182 Adams Avenue
San Diego, CA 92116
Voice: 619-281-7165
Web: www.autism.com/ari
A nonprofit organization whose purpose is to conduct research
  on autism and distribute its findings to parents and medical
  personnel.

Centers for Disease Control and Prevention
1600 Clifton Road
Atlanta, GA 30333
Hotline: 800-232-2522
Voice: 404-639-3311
Web: www.cdc.gov
A government organization that provides many opportunities to get
information about vaccines, including the following Web sites:
CDC Vaccine Safety: www.cdc.gov/nip/vacsafe
CDC Vaccines for Children Web site: www.cdc.gov/nip.vfc
CDC National Vaccine Program Office: www.cdc.gov/od/nvpo
Vaccine Price List: www.cdc.gov/nip/vfc/cdc_vaccine_price_list
.htm

Children's Defense Fund
25 E Street, NW
Washington, DC 20001
Voice: 202-628-8787
Web: www.childrensdefense.org
Mission: to Leave No Child Behind and to ensure every child a
Healthy Start, a Head Start, a Fair Start, a Safe Start, and a
Moral Start.

Food and Drug Administration
5600 Fishers Lane, HFI-40
Rockville, MD 20857
Voice: 888-463-6332
Web: www.fda.gov
E-mail: webmail@oc.fda.gov
Access the *FDA Consumer* magazine, as well as information about
immunization and vaccines.

Health Resources and Services Administration
1815 Fort Meyer Drive, Suite 300
Arlington, VA 22209

Voice: 703-908-9111
Web: www.hrsa.gov
E-mail: comments@hrsa.gov
Provides publications, resources, and referrals on health care services for low-income, uninsured individuals, and those with special health care needs.

Infectious Diseases Society of America
11 Canal Center Plaza, Suite 104
Alexandria, VA 22314
Voice: 703-200-0200
Web: www.idsociety.org
E-mail: info@idsociety.org
Provides information on immunizations, including a regular feature, "Immunization Newsbriefs."

Insure.com
Web: www.insure.com
A comprehensive site where you can ask questions about insurance coverage concerning vaccines.

Juvenile Diabetes Foundation
Web: www.jdf.org
Provides information about juvenile diabetes plus access to its magazine, *Countdown*.

National Institutes of Health (NIH)
9000 Rockville Pike
Bethesda, MD 20892
Voice: 301-496-4000
Web: www.nih.gov
Provides access to fact sheets, press releases, and clinical trial information regarding vaccines.

ORGANIZATIONS AND WEB SITES SPECIFICALLY RELATED TO VACCINES

This list includes government and nonprofit groups, organizations, and Web sites, including many parents' and citizens' groups, whose primary purpose is related to vaccines and immunizations.

Arizona Vaccine Information Network
Web: www.azavenue.com/kelly/organizations.htm
An excellent Web site for vaccine resources on all sides of the
    issue. More than five hundred resources listed for every aspect
    of vaccines and immunizations, from information on aborted
    tissue used in vaccines, to how to write a letter to get a religious
    exemption, to basic facts on vaccines. Also provides names of
    forums for parents with children harmed by vaccines.

Coalition for SAFE MINDs
Sensible Action for Ending Mercury-Induced Neurological Disorders
14 Commerce Drive, 3rd Floor
Cranford, NJ 07016
Voice: 908-276-8032

Every Child By Two
666 11th Street, NW, Suite 202
Washington, DC 20001
Voice: 202-783-7035
Web: www.ecbt.org
E-mail: info@ecbt.org
Their message is: "Shots by two if they're important to you." The
    Web site includes links to information and pictures of vaccine-
    preventable diseases.

Generation Rescue
Web: www.generationrescue.com
Information and resources for treating autism.

Global Vaccine Awareness League
PO Box 846
Lake Forest, CA 92630
Voice: 949-929-1191
Web: www.gval.com/index.html
Provides lists of states that allow medical, philosophical, and
religious exemptions as well as facts about vaccinations.

HealthWorld Information from Randall Neustaedter, O.M.D.
Web: www.healthy.net/vaccine

Immunization Action Coalition & The Hepatitis B Coalition
1573 Selby Avenue
St. Paul, MN 55104
Voice: 651-647-9009
Web: www.immunize.org
E-mail: admin@immunize.org
Purpose: to boost immunization rates and prevent disease.

Informed Parents Against VAPP (Vaccine-Associated Paralytic Polio)
PO Box 53212
Washington, DC 20009
Voice: 888-363-8277
Web: www.ipav.org
Pro-vaccination, pro–safe polio vaccines. This parents group seeks to
eliminate VAPP through advocacy efforts.

Institute for Vaccine Safety
Johns Hopkins School of Public Health
615 North Wolfe Street, Suite W5515
Baltimore, MD 21207
Voice: 410-995-2955
Web: www.vaccinesafety.edu
E-mail: info@vaccinesafety.edu

Provides links to information on current vaccine issues and
congressional testimony.

National Childhood Vaccine Injury Compensation Program
Parklawn Building, Room 8A-46
5600 Fishers Lane
Rockville, MD 20857
Voice: 301-443-6593; toll-free 800-338-2382
Web: www.hrsa.gov/bhpr/vicp
Provides access to the Vaccine Injury Table and information about
the National Vaccine Injury Compensation Program, how to file a
claim, and frequently asked questions.

National Network for Immunization Information (NNII)
Web: www.immunizationinfo.org
Mission: "To provide the public, health professionals, policy makers,
and the media with up to date, scientifically valid information
related to immunization to help them understand the issues and
to make informed decisions." This site is run by the Infectious
Diseases Society of America, the Pediatric Infectious Diseases
Society, the American Academy of Pediatrics, and the American
Nurses Association, and is funded by the Robert Wood Johnson
Foundation.

National Vaccine Information Center (NVIC)
512 West Maple Avenue, Suite 206
Vienna, VA 22180
Voice: 800-909-SHOT
Web: www.909shot.com
E-mail: info@909shot.com
Largest and oldest national, nonprofit educational organization
dedicated to preventing vaccine injuries and deaths through
public education. Many resources for parents concerned about
vaccine safety. Operates Vaccine Reaction Registry.

People Advocating Vaccine Education (PAVE)
Web: www.vaccines.bizland.com
Mission: "To help the public make informed and intelligent
    decisions about childhood and adult vaccines."

PKIDS—Parents of Kids with Infectious Diseases
PO Box 5666
Vancouver, WA 98668
Voice: 360-695-0293; toll-free 877-55-PKIDS
Web: www.pkids.org
E-mail: pkids@pkids.org
Provides information on immunizations, ask the experts,
    immunization table, search feature.

PROVE (Parents Requesting Open Vaccine Education)
Web: http://home.swbell.net/prove

Thinktwice Global Vaccine Institute
PO Box 9638-A
Santa Fe, NM 87504
Voice: 505-983-1856
Web: http://thinktwice.com/global.htm
Provides information you're not likely to get through mainstream
    sources.

Vaccine Adverse Events Reporting System (VAERS)
Voice: 800-822-7967
Web: www.fda.gov/cber/vaers/vaers.htm
Provides information about VAERS, how to report to them, the
    Table of Reportable Events, the Vaccine Injury Table, and other
    relevant material.

Vaccine Information & Awareness
Voice: 619-339-5498
Web: www.access1.net/via

E-mail: via@access1.net

Empowers parents to question, challenge, investigate, research, and become more informed and aware about vaccination risks and dangers that exist. Its major philosophical goal is to ensure that freedom of choice is not taken away from parents.

Vaccine Page: Vaccine News & Database
Web: www.vaccines.com
Assembled and run by the editors of UniScience News Net and supported in part by the Bill and Melinda Gates Children's Vaccine Program.

Vaccines: Are They Really Safe?
Web: www.garynull.com/Documents/vaccinesOverview.htm
A Web site by best-selling author Gary Null, PhD, that discusses specific vaccines and probes the health, economic, legal, and political factors surrounding vaccinations.

Vaccines Made from Aborted Babies
Web: www.dgwsoft.co.uk/homepages/vaccines/index.html
This site provides information on vaccines that are manufactured using cells derived from aborted fetuses and discusses the ethical issues.

VaccineWebsite.com
Web: www.whale.to/vaccines.html
Lots of links, articles, and other information about vaccines.

Glossary

❀

AAP: American Academy of Pediatrics. Among its many services, it helps determine vaccine schedules, safety, and efficacy.

ACIP: The Advisory Committee on Immunization Practices, part of the CDC. It recommends which vaccines should be on the Childhood Immunization Schedule.

AIDS (acquired immunodeficiency syndrome): The late stage of human immunodeficiency virus (HIV), characterized by a breakdown of the immune system and susceptibility to infections.

antibody: A protein molecule that identifies, neutralizes, and helps destroy pathogens (viruses, bacteria, fungi) and toxins. Antibodies are also known as immunoglobulins and are produced by cells called B lymphocytes when they are stimulated by antigens.

antigen: A substance, such as a bacterium, virus, or parasite, that induces the production of antibodies.

arthralgia: General term for mild to severe pain in the joints.

arthritis: General term for disease mainly characterized by inflammation of one or more joints, swelling, redness, stiffness, pain, and tenderness, especially with movement.

aseptic meningitis: Inflammation of the membranes that cover the spinal cord and brain. It is usually caused by a virus and creates flu-like symptoms, as well as severe headache, stiff neck, and stiffness in the spine. Most people recover completely within two weeks. Very severe cases can result in permanent muscle weakness or recurring bouts of aseptic meningitis. Symptoms of aseptic meningitis are similar to those of nonparalytic polio.

asthma: A respiratory disease in which the bronchial tubes become very irritated and the air passages narrow, resulting in difficulty breathing, wheezing, coughing, and production of thick mucus.

attention deficit disorder (ADD): A disorder characterized by an inability to sustain attention. Children typically are restless and easily frustrated and distracted.

attenuated: Weakened. Attenuated, or weakened, viruses are used in some vaccines because they can stimulate a strong immune response but do not cause the disease.

autism: A disorder, typically diagnosed before the age of three years, in which children isolate themselves from the outside world. Autistic children usually have little or no speech, refuse to make eye contact, engage in obsessive and repetitive behaviors such as head banging, spinning, and arm flapping, and are unable to relate emotionally to others.

autoimmune disease: A condition that is the result of the body attacking parts of itself, such as an organ, the joints, or tissue. In asthma, for example, the body attacks the bronchial tubes and air passages in the lungs.

booster: One or more vaccine doses given after the main dose(s) to increase the immune response to the components in the original vaccine dose(s).

CDC: The Centers for Disease Control and Prevention is involved in determining the safety and efficacy of vaccines. It has a National Immunization Program that answers questions about immunization from the public.

Crohn's disease: A chronic inflammatory disease of the intestinal tract characterized by abdominal pain, fever, loss of appetite, recurrent diarrhea, and weight loss. Anemia, stunted growth, and arthritis may occur, especially in children.

DNA (deoxyribonucleic acid): A double-stranded chain of molecules located in the nucleus of cells. It contains the genetic information that allows cells to reproduce and function.

DTaP: The diphtheria/tetanus/acellular pertussis vaccine.

encephalitis: Believed to be caused by a virus, this disorder is characterized by inflammation of the brain, which causes it to swell. Symptoms include personality changes, seizures, severe headache, confusion, partial paralysis, and alternating consciousness. Very severe cases can lead to coma and death. Many people recover without any permanent damage.

encephalopathy: A disease of the brain that can be caused by encephalitis, meningitis, seizures, trauma to the head, metabolic diseases, or other illnesses that affect the brain. Signs are similar to those of encephalitis.

enzyme: A protein that accelerates a chemical reaction without changing its own makeup.

epidemiology: The study of the frequency and distribution of disease in a given population.

FDA: The Food and Drug Administration. It can provide information to consumers about side effects associated with vaccinations.

Guillain-Barré syndrome: A rapidly progressing disease that affects the peripheral nervous system. It is characterized by muscle weakness, pain, paralysis, and numbness, typically starting in both legs and sometimes moving to the arms. More than 50 percent of people with GBS also have facial paralysis that may involve the tongue and eyes.

herpes zoster: Also known as shingles, this disorder is caused by the varicella zoster virus, the same virus that causes chicken pox. Herpes zoster is a very painful skin condition that can take up to four weeks to resolve. Older adults may suffer with complications such as fever, meningitis, vomiting, and neuralgia (nerve pain).

immunity: The natural or acquired ability of the immune system to resist disease. Immunity can be temporary or lifelong, specific to certain diseases, complete, or partial.

immunization: The administration of a vaccine to prompt the immune system to prevent infections when the body encounters them.

insulin-dependent diabetes mellitus (IDDM): Also known as juvenile diabetes or type 1 diabetes, IDDM is a chronic autoimmune disease in which the body cannot produce insulin and therefore cannot metabolize sugar (glucose).

interferon: A chemical produced by white blood cells that helps the body resist infections.

IPV: Inactivated polio vaccine.

learning disabilities: For the purpose of funding special-education programs, the federal government has defined *learning disability* as a disorder "in understanding or using language, spoken or written," that may appear as an "imperfect ability to listen, think, speak, read, write, spell or do mathematical calculations." Learning disabilities are believed to have many causes, including but not limited to genetic factors, biochemical abnormalities, bacterial and viral diseases, and other assaults to the central nervous system during early development.

MMR: The measles/mumps/rubella vaccine.

myelin sheath: A coating that covers the nerves and facilitates the transmission of signals between nerve cells.

NCVICP: The National Childhood Vaccine Injury Compensation Program provides complete information on how to file a claim for injuries associated with vaccinations.

neuropathy: Any functional disturbance or change in the peripheral nervous system, such as loss of sensation in the hands, feet, or face; muscle weakness or paralysis.

NVIC: National Vaccine Information Center. Provides information for parents about possible dangers associated with vaccine use and helps parents whose children have health problems believed to have been caused by vaccines.

OPV: Oral polio vaccine.

orchitis: Inflammation of the testes that occurs during or after mumps infection. Orchitis is usually accompanied by painful testes, high fever, nausea, vomiting, and headache. Approximately 20 to 35 percent of males get orchitis when they get the mumps, but sterility is very rare.

placebo: An inactive substance given to some participants in a study as a basis for comparison.

polyvalent vaccine: A vaccine that contains multiple viral strains or that is made to induce immune responses against multiple strains.

RNA (ribonucleic acid): A single-stranded molecule that carries genetic information.

seizures: Convulsions—involuntary contractions of the muscles caused by a disturbance in the electrical activity of the brain. There are many different types of seizures, and they can last for several seconds up to several hours.

subacute sclerosing panencephalitis (SSPE): A rare, fatal disease that affects children and adolescents. It is believed to be caused by a viral infection, specifically an atypical measles virus or one closely related to measles virus. It is a slowly progressive disease: It can take one year or more between the time a person is exposed to the measles virus and the appearance of symptoms of SSPE.

subunit vaccine: Also referred to as recombinant vaccines, subunit vaccines contain only a part of the virus or other organisms rather than the whole organism.

sudden infant death syndrome (SIDS): Sometimes referred to as crib death, SIDS is the sudden, unexplained death of an apparently healthy child. Death usually occurs between the ages of two weeks and one year, with the peak occurring between two and four months of age. Nearly every death occurs when the child is sleeping.

thrombocytopenia purpura: An autoimmune disorder characterized by a reduction in the number of platelets circulating in the bloodstream. This thinned blood seeps into the tissues under the skin, causing blotchy red patches on the body.

titer: A measure of the amount or concentration of a substance in a solution—for example, the concentration of antibodies for rubella in the bloodstream.

vaccine: A preparation that stimulates an immune response that can create resistance to or prevent infection.

VAERS: The Vaccine Adverse Events Reporting System is a program created by the FDA and CDC to receive and analyze reports of adverse reactions to vaccines.

virus: A microorganism that consists of RNA or DNA surrounded by protein. It reproduces by infecting a cell and making the cell's components produce new viruses.

Suggested Reading List

❁

Bock, Kenneth, and Cameron Stauth, *Healing the New Childhood Epidemics: Autism, ADHD, Asthma, Allergies: The Groundbreaking Program for the 4-A Disorders,* New York, NY: Ballantine Books, 2008.

Compart, Pamela, and Dana Laake, *The Kid-Friendly ADHD and Autism Cookbook: The Ultimate Guide to the Gluten-Free, Casein-Free Diet,* Beverly, MA: Fair Winds Press, 2006.

Coulter, Harris L., and Barbara Loe Fisher, *A Shot in the Dark: Why the P in the DPT Vaccination May Be Hazardous to Your Child's Health,* New York, NY: Avery Trade Publishing, 1991. Written by a medical historian (Coulter) and the president of the National Vaccine Information Center (Fisher), this book documents the risks associated with the DPT vaccine.

Edelson, Stephen, and Bernard Rimland, editors, *Recovering Autistic Children,* San Diego, CA: Autism Research Institute, 2006.

Jepson, Bryan, Katie Wright, and Jane Johnson, *Changing the Course of Autism: A Scientific Approach for Parents and Physicians,* Boulder, CO: Sentient Publications, 2007.

Kirby, David, *Evidence of Harm: Mercury in Vaccines and the Autism Epidemic,* New York, NY: St. Martin's Press, 2006.

Lewis, Lisa, *Special Diets for Special People: Understanding and Implementing a Gluten-Free and Casein-Free Diet to Aid in the Treatment of Autism and Related Developmental Disorders,* Arlington, TX: Future Horizons Press, 2005.

Lewis, Lisa, and Karyn Seroussi, *The Encyclopedia of Dietary In-*

terventions for the Treatment of Autism and Related Disorders, Pennington, NJ: Sarpsborg Press, 2008.

McCandless, Jaquelyn, *Children with Starving Brains,* Putney, VT: Bramble Books, 2007.

McCarthy, Jenny, *Louder Than Words: A Mother's Journey in Healing Autism,* New York, NY: Dutton, 2007.

Miller, Neil Z., *Vaccines: Are They Really Safe and Effective?* Santa Fe, NM: New Atlantean Press, 2008.

————, *Vaccine Safety Manual for Concerned Families and Health Practitioners: Guide to Immunization Risks and Protection,* Santa Fe, NM: New Atlantean Press, 2008.

Neustaedter, Randall, *The Vaccine Guide: Risks and Benefits for Children and Adults,* Berkeley, CA: North Atlantic Books, 2002.

Pangborn, Jon, and Sidney MacDonald Baker, *Autism: Effective Biomedical Treatments (Have We Done Everything We Can for This Child? Individuality in an Epidemic),* San Diego, CA: Autism Research Institute, 2005.

Sears, Robert, *The Vaccine Book: Making the Right Decision for Your Child,* New York, NY: Little, Brown and Company, 2007.

Seroussi, Karyn, *Unraveling the Mystery of Autism and Pervasive Developmental Disorder: A Mother's Story of Research and Recovery,* New York, NY: Broadway Books, 2000.

Tenpenny, Sherri, *Vaccines: The Risks, the Benefits, the Choices, A Resource Guide for Parents,* Sevierville, TN: Insight Publishing, 2006.

Index

ABOUT THE AUTHOR

Stephanie Cave, M.D., was born in New Orleans, Louisiana. She received a BS in medical technology from Louisiana State University in 1966, an MS in clinical chemistry from Louisiana State University Medical School in 1978, and an M.D. from Louisiana State University Medical School in 1983. She completed a residency in family medicine and is on the clinical faculty at Louisiana State University Medical School. She has been in private practice since 1986. She is board-certified in family practice and is a fellow of the American Academy of Family Physicians. Married to attorney Donald Cave, she has three sons and ten grandchildren. Since 1995, Dr. Cave has treated more than nine thousand children in the autism spectrum. Having testified before the congressional Committee on Governmental Reform in 2000 regarding mercury in vaccines, she has traveled extensively lecturing on autism, vaccines, and the clinical aspects of mercury toxicity.